BLENDER SHOWROOM

This section will do a quick breakdown of our overall impression of some of the most popular blenders on the market. We take into account the quality of the motor & blade, ease of use, and overall quality of food that is produced by each machine.
Some people use blenders only for smoothies and others for crushing ice and making simple liquids and spreads. More advanced cooks use them to mill grains, making hot soups and purees, even kneading dough and making batter.

HIGH-END BLENDERS

Vitamix:

If you can shell out for the hefty $650 price tag, the Vitamix blender takes home the gold trophy. It is one seriously high-powered blender that can do it all -- there is literally no limit to what you can do with this machine.

Pros:
● blends just about anything
● grind nuts and seeds -- completely breaking apart cell walls, turning them to dust
● smash frozen fruit into a soft cream
● warm up soups, sauces and dips by spinning them at a whopping 240 mph
● 7 year warranty

Cons:
● giant price tag
Side note: You can purchase a "factory reconditioned" machine for around $299 at their website. You basically get a refurbished model that is certified to work like a brand new one for nearly half the price!

Blendtec

A worthy rival to the Vitamix, it is also slightly more cost-effective than the Vitamix. Surprisingly, its actually a little more powerful with its 1560 watt machine (compared to Vitamix's 1380 watts).

Pros:
● easy to clean and get out food that is trapped under the blades.
● super powerful motor
● warms up pretty much any liquid

Cons:
● does not come with a tamper -- a tool used to push food into the blades
● cannot fill the pitcher all the way to the top and expect perfect blending
● can be louder than the Vitamix when blending

Nutribullet

A more recent contender in the high-speed blender market, it has quickly risen to fame for what it can do with its cheaper price tag (you can get one for $90-130). This machine comes at 600 watts, which is half the power of the Vitamix or Blendtec.

Pros:
- great price tag for what you get
- can grind nuts, grains and seeds
- can make most things as its opponents, but you just have to be more patient

Cons:
- the pitcher is only 24oz, so expect to make smaller quantities at a time
- its shelf life is questionable at best

Ninja Blender

Another popular contender in the blender market, this one tends to be more affordable. It comes with multiple blades, unlike any of the others we featured in our showroom, and eliminates the need for a tamper. It's spectacular design even features blades in the middle and top -- which is hard to find anywhere else.
This one is comparable to the Nutribullet, thus, if you are patient, you can achieve a lot with this blender for the price. That means you should expect to re-blend certain recipes a few times to achieve great results.

Pros:
- much more affordable blender
- can make decent liquid foods
- great for making smoothies
- great for large amounts of liquids
- suitable for households with multiple people

Cons:
- not the strongest blender

DRINK SMOOTHIES TO FEEL INCREDIBLE & LOOK SEXY

1.   **Easily consume fruits and vegetables**. Most people struggle to get their daily recommended dose of nutrients, so they resort to artificial methods such as pills and gummies. Smoothies are a fantastic way to nourish your body the most natural way possible -- fresh fruits and vegetables.
2.   **So easy to make.** With a decent blender, you can quickly and effortlessly throw in fresh ingredients, blend, and be out the kitchen in under 5 minutes. So no excuses even for the busiest people.
3.   **Easy weight loss.** Drop the extra weight without any extra effort by feeding your body the essential nutrients it needs, while satisfying your craving for sweet or savory foods. By using naturally sweet ingredients like honey, you can easily cut out the heavily-

4.   **Supercharge your energy and reduce cravings.** Because smoothies are basically pure nutrition (barring any sweeteners you add), you will feel a surge of energy when you consistently feed your body natural fuel. This depends from person to person how long it takes to feel this way since some people's bodies need to readjust from processing garbage to natural foods. If you keep up these positive habits, your body will certainly reverse those old bad ones and start appreciating you for eating only high quality food. The best part is that you will also be less hungry often since you are satiating the internal systems with way fewer calories.

5.   **Superior digestion and nutrient absorption.** Imagine how much chewing you would have to get through to swallow a plate of veggies and fruits. Let the blender do the work for you and easily gulp down all the natural fiber-y goodness to jumpstart your digestive processes. It takes a lot of effort to efficiently break down the foods you normally chew and swallow. You are actually allowing your body to more effectively absorb the nutrients you just fed it.

6.   **Easy way to detox.** We bombard our bodies with countless artificial chemicals on a daily basis. These chemicals are called "free-radicals" and basically travel freely through your body, sometimes attaching to other chemicals to create new dangerous compounds (this is one way certain cancers form). Now you can easily introduce wonderful antioxidants that clear out these terrible toxins.

7.   **Infinite options for flavor.** Because there are so many fruits, vegetables, spices and herbs, supplements, oils and fats, there is literally no limit to how many types of smoothies you can create. Seriously, how amazing is that? If you can't stand drinking the same thing everyday, this is a great way for you to mix up your meal plans. You will get excited about trying new things

8.   **Feel sexy with gorgeous skin, hair and nails.** The influx of vitamins and minerals in your diet will have noticeable effects on the outside of your body also, not just your internal organ systems. If you drink smoothies regularly, you can expect your skin, hair and nails to glow radiantly and catch the attention of everyone around you.

9.   **Stop getting sick.** You are equipping your body's natural defenses with an entire army of vitamins and minerals to literally destroy foreign substances that cause sickness.

10. **Overall happiness.** This one is the most endearing benefit you will experience. Because your body's overall functions -- that means everything from the inside to outside -- are working at their optimal levels, you will feel much more calm and happy for no "specific" reason.

Juicing vs Blending: What's The Difference?

While the answer to this question might be obvious to some, most people don't understand that there is, in fact, a clear difference between juicing and blending.

The easiest way to clear the confusion is to focus on one major quality in taste and consistency that differs between juices and smoothies. When juicing, the machine is extracting the water and the majority of the nutrients the produce contains -- but leaves the pulp behind. Blenders, on the other hand, smash every juicy bit and piece of the produce to create a thicker and fuller consistency (keeping the insoluble fiber that is also good for you).

This leaves only one more question on the table. Which is better for you?

The answer to this question will depend on your health goals. While both are great choices, just keep a few things in mind:

● Because juice retains only soluble fiber, nutrients pass through your system much more quickly (easy digestion)

● Smoothies will keep you full longer since digesting them takes a little longer

● You can easily consume more produce when juicing (but that means no thick fruits like bananas or avocados)

Tips & Techniques

How To Save 10+ Hours A Week

So you want to start a smoothie diet. Whether you want to lose weight, feel incredibly energetic, or just consume more natural vitamins and minerals, drinking a delicious smoothie doesn't have to be hard. It doesn't even have to take longer than 10 minutes! If you're sick of processed foods and chemical-laced junk, then start enjoying nutritious, well-balanced beverages. You'll love how sexy you look and feel when you start a natural diet.

Whatever your reasons, you're reading this book because:

A. you own a blender, and

B. you have no time to cook.

We understand. We're here for you. We want to help.

Sometimes, it seems like no amount of preparation or whole nights spent in our kitchens will get us anywhere. So much planning and cooking, and for what? An okay meal, and a really big mess. Not anymore! In this book, we'll help you:

● Plan shopping ahead, with a list of the must-have ingredients for the majority of the recipes found in this book.

● Get in the habit of planning and freezing for easy, nearly no-chopping meal preparation.

● Follow recipes for new and amazingly simple dishes that you'll love, and that require no more than a couple free hours on a Sunday or some free time in the morning.

Freeze N' Throw

To make your preparation time in the mornings even shorter, set aside ten minutes each weekend to plan ahead your shopping list (for any ingredients that you don't already have ready). This way, you won't be frazzled Monday morning when, halfway through a recipe, you realize you don't have any coconut milk. It's the worst. We've all done it.

To make things even easier on yourself, go ahead and chop up the veggies that you'll need for the week and freeze them! Whether in plastic baggies or re-sealable plastic containers, it'll be a breeze in the mornings to take what you need out of the freezer, measure it out, and throw it in the slow cooker. That's it!

While some recipes call for "one whole diced onion" or "half of a green pepper", just remember: roughly, a whole pepper or small/medium onion is one cup. When it comes to garlic, one clove is roughly one teaspoon, minced. Over time, you'll become comfortable with eyeballing and knowing how much or how little to use.

Even if you throw in a few more pre-chopped carrots or celery than a recipe calls for, what's the hurt? Extra veggies are always a good thing! Cooking can be a wonderful way to experiment and learn about flavors and measurements, and there's no easier way to cook than blending.

Now, all that's left to do is start! Life is busy and chaotic, but cooking dinner doesn't have to be. With a little planning, a little tossing, and a lot of delicious and satisfying meals, drinking smoothies won't be difficult ever again.

Fruits	Vegetables	Nuts, Herbs, Oils & Toppings	Liquids
Blueberries	Spinach		Coconut milk
Bananas	Kale	Greek yogurt	almond milk
Avocados	Celery	almond butter	Coconut water
Apples (red & green)	Carrots	Peanut butter	
Strawberries	Ginger	Coconut oil	
Pineapples	Beets	Walnuts	
Lemons	Cucumbers	almonds	
Peaches	Broccoli	Honey	
Oranges	Beans	Cinnamon	
Limes	Romaine lettuce	Turmeric	
Raspberry		Chili powder	
Tomatoes		Flax seeds	
Grapes			
Kiwis		Cayenne pepper	
Dates		Cilantro	
		Agave nectar	
		Honey	
		Basil	
		Parsley	
		Cumin	
		butter	
		Shredded cheese	
		Dried oregano	
		Cayenne pepper	
		Thyme	

SUPERFOOD GUIDE

Simply put, a superfood is a nutrient-rich substance that is thought to be especially beneficial to health. This list is here to help you make quick decisions about what ingredients to include in your grocery list, but is by no means a comprehensive or exclusive list.

1. **Greek yogurt** -- a thicker and creamier yogurt that has a higher concentration of protein than regular yogurt
2. **Blueberries** -- loaded with vitamin C and powerful antioxidants
3. **Cranberries** -- help fight inflammation and full of antioxidants and vitamin C
4. **Acai berry --** one of the fruits known to be richest in antioxidants
5. **Strawberries** -- loaded with vitamin C and antioxidants
6. **Flax seeds** -- loaded with omega-3's and lignans that help prevent cancer
7. **Chia seeds** -- contain high amounts of essential fatty acids, magnesium, iron, calcium, and potassium

8.   **Kale** -- a bitter green leaf chock full of fiber, calcium, iron, and antioxidants
9.   **Broccoli** -- a very mean green that packs a powerful punch of vitamins, minerals, and fiber
10. **Spinach** -- a superior green leaf that contains high amounts of antioxidants, anti-inflammatories, and vitamins to promote many basic functions (including eye and bone development)
11. **Almonds** -- a very nutrient-dense nut that is loaded with calcium, vitamin E, magnesium, and iron
12. **Ginger** -- more common in Asian cooking, ginger is world-renowned for its anti-inflammatory properties
13. **Carrots** -- world-renowned to fight cardiovascular disease and improve vision systems in the body
14. **Coconut** -- loaded with a unique chain of fatty acids that have powerful positive effects on health, including improved brain function
15. **Dark chocolate** -- celebrate that this substance is loaded with nutrients from the cacao tree, including powerful antioxidants and iron, magnesium, copper, and manganese

VITAMIX QUICKSTART GUIDE:

ZERO TO HERO IN 10 MIN OR LESS

To get the most out your blender, keep it in a dedicated place in your kitchen. Think of this as your smoothie station, not that smoothies are all you can make with this fantastic device.

If you are new to the Vitamix, here are some basic rules you MUST remember if you don't want to break your machine:

Adding some liquid (such as water) will make blending much easier and preserve the life of your blades.

Most recipes are completely blended within 60 seconds. If you need to blend a little more, try using the tamper to push the chunkier items from the top of the pitcher to the bottom.
If the motor stops working, you MUST unplug the base and let the machine cool for at least an hour before trying to use it again.

Make sure that the cord is conveniently stashed away and not exposed to hot surfaces, as this will cause it to melt.

Certain fruits have seeds and pits that will release dangerous cyanide into your drinks (usually in small amounts, but daily use can cause serious damage). Some examples are: apple seeds, cherry pits, peach pits, plum pits, apricot pits, etc.

There is an optimal way to load the pitcher for easy blending. See image below.

HOW TO USE PARTS CORRECTLY

40 OZ CONTAINER:

- Perfect for blending in large quantities
- Use for thick mixtures and hot **ingredients**
- Unplug lid to:
•add ingredients to create layered textures (like chunky tomatoes in tomato soup)
•use tamper to push food down

20 OZ CONTAINER:

- Perfect for blending individual beverages
- Great for chopping ingredients or emulsifying vinaigrettes
- Use to maintain temperature of individual beverages on the go
- Can add flip-top lid to carry with you

TAMPER:

- Use to help frozen or thick mixtures circulate better
- Remove lid plug while machine is running and insert tamper through hole

- Move tamper in circles in container to push ingredients into the blades
- The lid is designed to prevent tamper from reaching the blades

EASY CLEANING TIPS

THE POWER BASE

The Power Base generally won't get dirty, but liquids can lead into it if the lid is not sealed tightly onto the cups. Unplug the base and wipe both the inside and outside with a damp cloth.

Do NOT submerge the base underwater, or attempt to clean it in the dishwasher. Seriously.

THE CONTAINERS

Cleaning the containers is dead simple. All you have to do is rinse out whatever food is remaining in the cup and wash it as you would any regular cup -- by hand or in the dishwasher.

If there are thick substances (like peanut butter) that are stuck in there and won't come out, one option is to fill the cup with ⅔ solution of soapy water and screw on the milling blade. Blend this soapy cocktail for about 20-30 seconds to loosen whatever is stuck inside, and rinse everything out.

Everything from the blade base and lids to the containers and seals (EXCEPT motor base) are dishwasher safe. It is highly recommended that you use only the top rack of the dishwasher since the bottom rack tends to generate the most heat and could potentially warp the plastic materials.

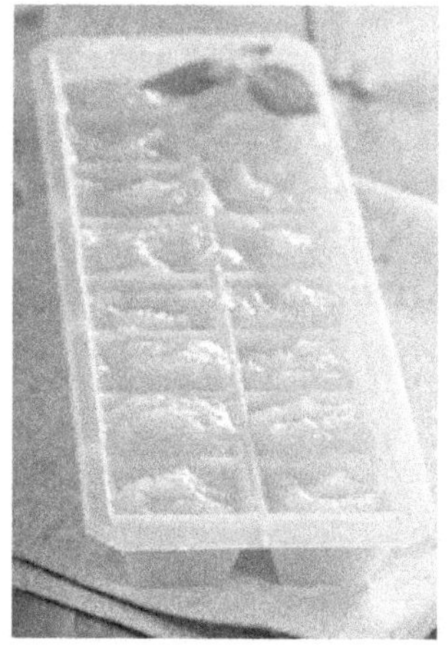

USE THE VITAMIX LIKE A PRO

Flavored ice cubes. You can easily replace regular ice cubes with flavored ones by freezing your favorite fruit juice or tea ahead of time. When it's time to make your smoothie, just throw in these flavored cubes for an enhanced flavor and texture -- while keeping it nice and cold.

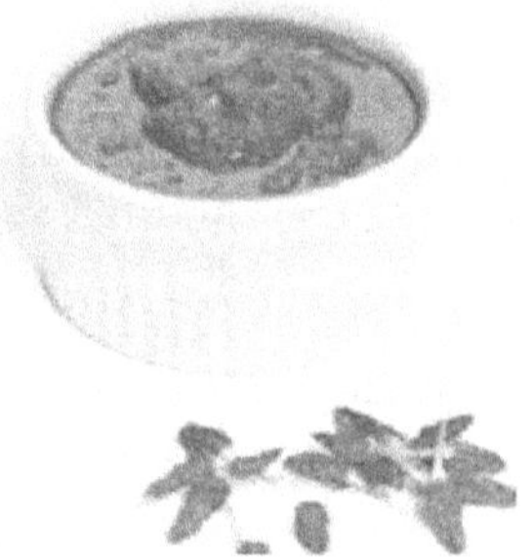

Quickly make dips, spreads, and salsas.

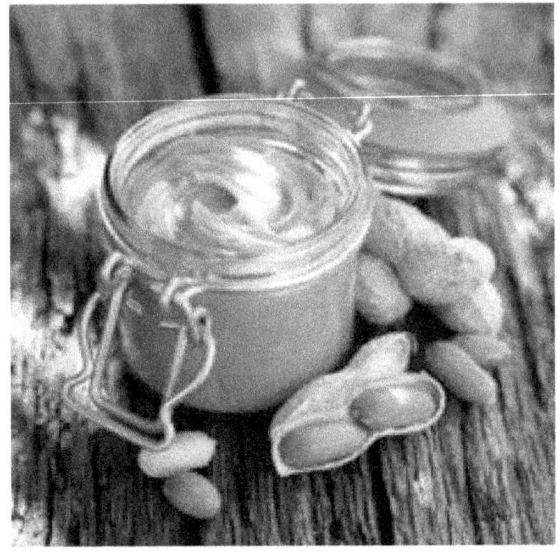

Store your creations in jars to preserve them longer.

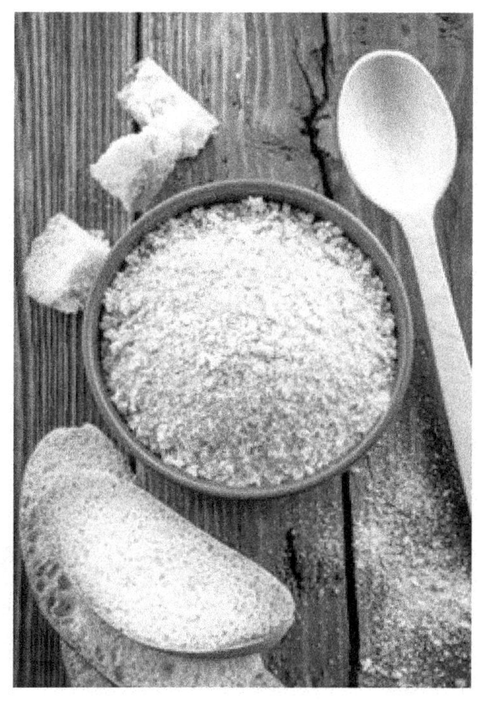

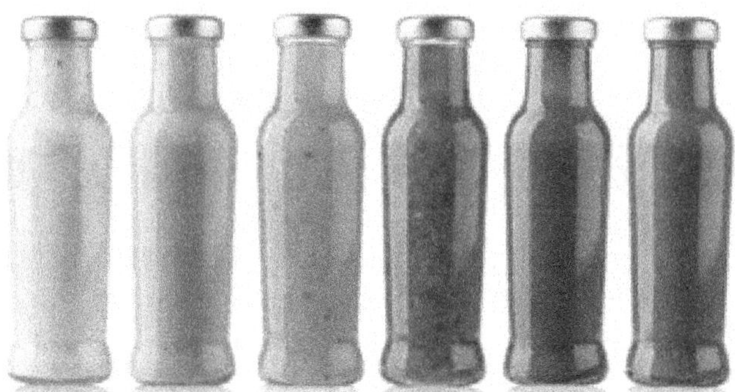

Easily make food crumbs for pies or as a topping.

Make different sauces and dressings to create a variety of flavors for all your meals throughout the week.

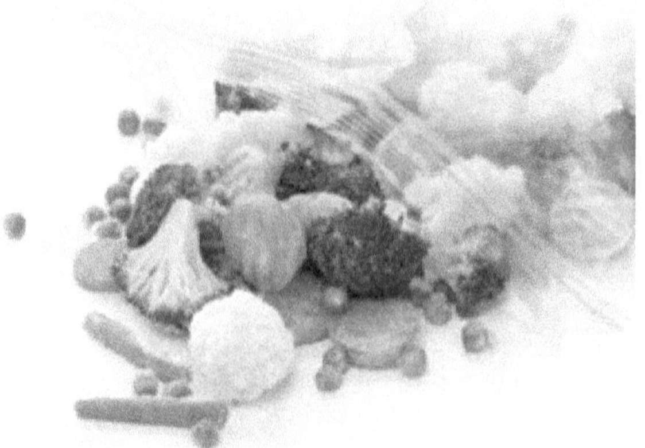

Store your chopped veggies and fruits in frozen bags to get in and out of the kitchen quickly.

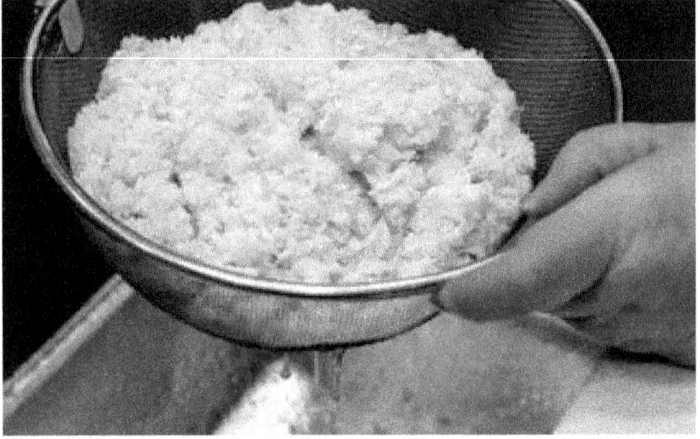

The best way to shred vegetables like cabbage without making them mushy is to add a little water to the container before processing.

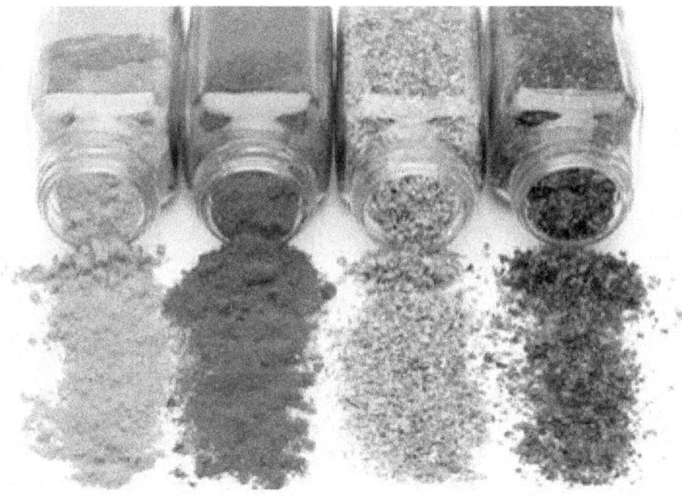

Create your own fresh herb spice blends for an infinite number of flavor combinations.

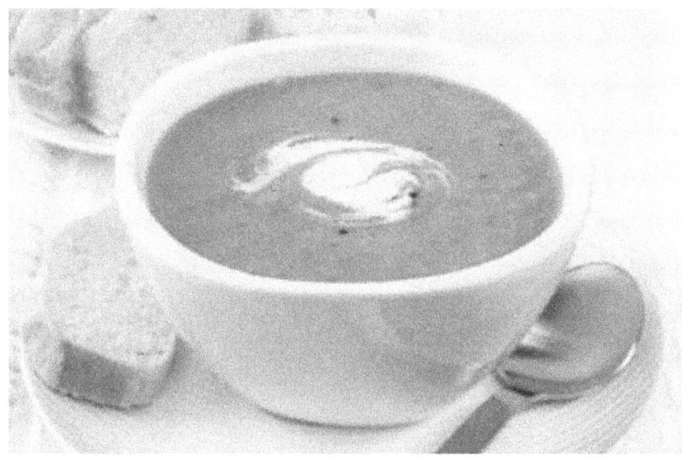

If you get bored of smoothies and juices, you can always make fresh soups that are equally nutritious.

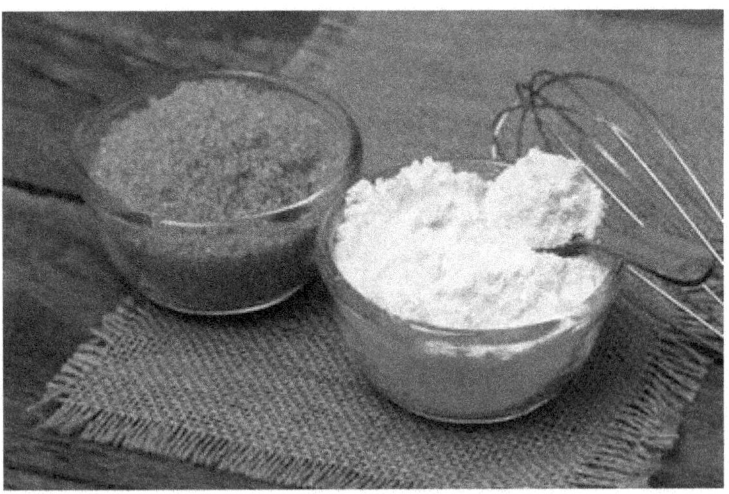

If you are going gluten-free, easily create low-gluten flour by grinding rice such as wild rice or brown rice (anything that is low- on the glycemic index is good)

RECIPES FOR TOTAL HEALTH REJUVENATION

100 SMOOTHIE RECIPES

Directions:
1.   Add liquid first, then softer ingredients and harder items like ice last.
2.   Blend on medium and increase to high for 1 minute.
Note: To create layered textures, slow down speed setting and add ingredients by unplugging lid and using the opening.

20 SUPERFOOD RECIPES

BLUEBERRY FLAX SUPERFOOD SMOOTHIE

Ingredients
1 cup blueberries, frozen
1 tbsp flaxseed, ground
Handful of spinach
¼ cup full-fat Greek yogurt
1 cup coconut milk or any kind of milk
Directions:
1.   Add liquid first, then softer ingredients and harder items like ice last.
2.   Blend on medium and increase to high for 1 minute. Repeat as necessary.

SUPERFOOD POWER SMOOTHIE

Ingredients
2 large bananas, previously peeled, sliced, and frozen
1 heaping handful spinach (about 1.5 cups)
1/2 of a large apple, chopped (or 1 small)
1/2 cup almond milk
1 tbsp ground flax (optional)
7 large strawberries, sliced
Directions:
1.   Add liquid first, then softer ingredients and harder items like ice last.
2.   Blend on medium and increase to high for 1 minute. Repeat as necessary.

MINT CHIP SUPERFOOD SMOOTHIE

Ingredients
2-3 frozen bananas
1-2 tbsps hemp milk or other non-dairy milk
1 tbsp hemp seeds
½ to 1 teaspoon spirulina powder
2 drops peppermint oil
1½ tbsps dark chocolate chips or cocoa nibs, divided
Directions:
1.   Add liquid first, then softer ingredients and harder items like ice last.
2.   Blend on medium and increase to high for 1 minute. Repeat as necessary.

MACA ALMOND CACAO SMOOTHIE

Ingredients
1/4 cup almond milk
2 frozen bananas
2 tbsps almond butter
1 date cacao beans/nibs
1 tbsp coconut oil
1 tbsp Maca
Directions:
1.   Add liquid first, then softer ingredients and harder items like ice last.

2. Blend on medium and increase to high for 1 minute. Repeat as necessary.

VEGAN SUPERFOOD CHOCOLATE SMOOTHIE

Ingredients
2 bananas
6 ice cubes
1 tbsp coconut oil
1 tbsp dairy free plain yogurt
1 tbsp chia seeds
2 tbsp hemp seeds
1 tsp camu camu powder
1 tsp cacao
¼ cup coconut milk (or unsweetened almond milk)
Directions:
1. Add liquid first, then softer ingredients and harder items like ice last.
2. Blend on medium and increase to high for 1 minute. Repeat as necessary.

AVOCADO SUPERFOOD SMOOTHIE

Ingredients
1 Hass avocado
1 1/2 cups frozen blueberries
3 strawberries
17 mint leaves
1 1/2 cups organic orange juice
1/4 cup plain yogurt
2 tbsps agave nectar
1/2 cup frozen raspberries
Directions:
1. Add liquid first, then softer ingredients and harder items like ice last.
2. Blend on medium and increase to high for 1 minute. Repeat as necessary.

GREEN COCONUT SMOOTHIE (HEALTHY)

Ingredients
2 bananas, frozen

2 big handfuls spinach
1 cup milk
1/4 teaspoon cinnamon
1 teaspoon vanilla
1 tbsp coconut oil
Directions:
1. Add liquid first, then softer ingredients and harder items like ice last.
2. Blend on medium and increase to high for 1 minute. Repeat as necessary.

BANANA BEET SMOOTHIE

Ingredients
2 bananas, frozen
1 medium sized golden beet
¼ cup rolled oats (optional)
1 cup unsweetened almond milk
1/2 cup full-fat coconut milk
½ teaspoon vanilla extract
Pinch cinnamon (optional)
Directions:
1. Add liquid first, then softer ingredients and harder items like ice last.
2. Blend on medium and increase to high for 1 minute. Repeat as necessary.

GREEN SMOOTHIE

Ingredients
1 cup hemp milk
1 cup kale packed
2 cups frozen pineapple
2 kiwis, whole
1/2 avocado
1 banana
1 T. coconut oil
1 T. maca powder
Directions:
1. Add liquid first, then softer ingredients and harder items like ice last.
2. Blend on medium and increase to high for 1 minute. Repeat as necessary.

BERRY BLAST ALMOND SMOOTHIE

Ingredients

1 cup unsweetened almond milk
¼ cup fat free vanilla Greek yogurt, or a dairy free yogurt
2 heaping tbsps protein powder
about 8 to 10 raw almonds
1 tbsp golden flax seeds
½ cup blueberries
5 or 6 strawberries
small handful of fresh spinach

Directions:

1.   Add liquid first, then softer ingredients and harder items like ice last.
2.   Blend on medium and increase to high for 1 minute. Repeat as necessary.

BLUEBERRY MANGO AND SUPERFOOD SMOOTHIE

Ingredients

200 ml organic goat or soy yogurt
1 handful frozen blueberries
1 handful frozen mango
1 tbsp bee pollen
1 tbs goji berries
1/2 cup of raw oats or almonds

Directions:

1.   Add liquid first, then softer ingredients and harder items like ice last.
2.   Blend on medium and increase to high for 1 minute. Repeat as necessary.

SUPERFOOD PB BANANA AND CACAO GREEN SMOOTHIE

Ingredients

3/4 cup unsweetened vanilla almond milk
1 loose cup baby spinach
2 teaspoons peanut butter
1/2 frozen ripe banana
1/3 oz (heaping tbsp) cacao nibs
1 cup ice
(optional) a few drops liquid Stevia

Directions:

1.   Add liquid first, then softer ingredients and harder items like ice last.
2.   Blend on medium and increase to high for 1 minute. Repeat as necessary.

SUPERFOOD PUMPKIN PIE SMOOTHIE

Ingredients

1 frozen banana
½ cup Greek yogurt
½ teaspoon pumpkin pie spice
½ cup almond milk
2 tbsps pure maple syrup
¼ teaspoon vanilla
⅔ cup pumpkin puree
1 tbsp flax seeds
1 cup ice

Directions:

1.   Add liquid first, then softer ingredients and harder items like ice last.
2.   Blend on medium and increase to high for 1 minute. Repeat as necessary.

SUPERFOOD CHIA GREEN SMOOTHIE

Ingredients

2 cups cold water
2 handfuls spinach
1 kale leaf, medium
1/2 long English cucumber, sliced
1/2 any apple, chopped and not cored/seeded/peeled
2 tbsp chia seeds
1/2 lemon, juice

Directions:

1.   Add liquid first, then softer ingredients and harder items like ice last.

2.   Blend on medium and increase to high for 1 minute. Repeat as necessary.

CHOCOLATE-CAULIFLOWER SMOOTHIE RECIPES FROM 'SUPERFOOD SMOOTHIES'

Ingredients
1/4 cup Medjool dates, pitted (about 3–4 large fruits)
3 cups steamed cauliflower
1/4 cup cacao nibs
2 tbsp hemp seeds
1 tbsp cacao powder
1 ½ cups rice milk, original variety
2 cups coconut ice
Sweetener, to taste
Directions:
1.   Add liquid first, then softer ingredients and harder items like ice last.
2.   Blend on medium and increase to high for 1 minute. Repeat as necessary.

SUPERFOOD TRIPLE BERRY CHIA PUDDING

Ingredients
1 cup unsweetened almond/coconut milk beverage
3/4 cup fresh blueberries, blackberries and raspberries
2 tbsp chia seeds
5-6 drops sugar/honey to taste
Directions:
1.   Add liquid first, then softer ingredients and harder items like ice last.
2.   Blend on medium and increase to high for 1 minute. Repeat as necessary.

CHOCOLATE MALT SUPERFOOD SMOOTHIE

Ingredients
2 frozen bananas
1½ tbsps maca root powder

1 tbsp raw cacao powder or 2 tbsps cocoa powder
1 medjool date, pitted
1 teaspoon pure vanilla extract
2-4 tbsps water
optional: cacao nibs
Directions:
1.   Add liquid first, then softer ingredients and harder items like ice last.
2.   Blend on medium and increase to high for 1 minute. Repeat as necessary.

EGGLESS NOG SUPERFOOD SMOOTHIE

Ingredients
2 tbsp superfood powder
1 cup Vanilla almond Milk
2 cups (1 large apple) Apple (chopped)
2 whole, pitted Date
1/4 tsp Nutmeg (ground)
1/2 tsp Vanilla Extract
1/4 cup Walnuts
1/4 cup Water
1.5 cups Ice
Directions:
1.   Add liquid first, then softer ingredients and harder items like ice last.
2.   Blend on medium and increase to high for 1 minute. Repeat as necessary.

SPICY CITRUS AND BERRY SMOOTHIE WITH CHIA SEEDS

Ingredients
1 ½ cups freshly squeezed orange juice
¼ cup pure mangosteen juice
1 ½ cups frozen red raspberries
1 ½ cups frozen peach slices
1 tbsp chia seeds
1 tbsp coconut oil, melted
Few pinches of cayenne pepper, to taste
Directions:

1.   Add liquid first, then softer ingredients and harder items like ice last.
2.   Blend on medium and increase to high for 1 minute. Repeat as necessary.

BLUEBERRY AVOCADO AND SPINACH SUPERFOOD SMOOTHIE

Ingredients
1 cup blueberries, frozen or fresh
1 cup fresh spinach leaves
1 cup almond-coconut milk
½ ripe avocado, skinned and pitted
1 tbsp chia seeds
¼ teaspoon cinnamon
1 tbsp honey
1 scoop protein powder
½ fresh ice
Directions:
3.   Add liquid first, then softer ingredients and harder items like ice last.
4.   Blend on medium and increase to high for 1 minute. Repeat as necessary.

20 HIGH-PROTEIN RECIPES

BANANA RASPBERRY CHIA SMOOTHIE

Ingredients
½ banana
½ cup raspberries
½ cup plain Greek yogurt
1 tbsp chia seeds
1 scoop protein powder
½ cup water
½ teaspoon cinnamon
pinch nutmeg
two handfuls ice - to taste
Directions:
1.   Add liquid first, then softer ingredients and harder items like ice last.
2.   Blend on medium and increase to high for 1 minute. Repeat as necessary.

STRAWBERRY BANANA SMOOTHIE WITH CHIA SEEDS

Ingredients
1 cup (250 mL) fresh strawberries, hulled and cleaned
1 peeled banana, frozen
4 cubes of ice
1 T chia seeds soaked in ¼ cup (60 mL) of water
⅓ cup (160 mL) light coconut milk
Directions:
1.   Add liquid first, then softer ingredients and harder items like ice last.
2.   Blend on medium and increase to high for 1 minute. Repeat as necessary.

BLUEBERRY MANGO SMOOTHIE

Ingredients
1 cup frozen blueberries
1 cup mango chunks
1 cup plain Greek yogurt
1/4 cup vanilla soy milk, almond milk, or skim milk or water
Directions:
1.   Add liquid first, then softer ingredients and harder items like ice last.
2.   Blend on medium and increase to high for 1 minute. Repeat as necessary.

PAPAYA GINGER SMOOTHIE

Ingredients
1 ½ cups papaya, chilled and cut into chunks
1 cup ice
½ cup nonfat plain Greek yogurt
2 teaspoons fresh ginger, peeled and chopped
Juice of half a lemon
1 teaspoon agave nectar
Leaves from one sprig of mint
Directions:
1.   Add liquid first, then softer ingredients and harder items like ice or frozen fruit last.
2.   Blend on medium and increase to high for 1 minute. Repeat as necessary.

PEANUT BUTTER AND JELLY PROTEIN SMOOTHIE

Ingredients
1 cup frozen berries
1 tbsp all-natural peanut butter
1 scoop Vanilla Bean, Designer Whey Sustained Energy
2 tbsps rolled oats
1 cup soy milk
Directions:
1.   Add liquid first, then softer ingredients and harder items like ice or frozen fruit last.

2.   Blend on medium and increase to high for 1 minute. Repeat as necessary.

FRENCH TOAST PROTEIN SHAKE

Ingredients
1/2 cup Fat free cottage cheese
11 Scoop vanilla protein powder
21 tsp Maple extract (or 2 tbs sugar free maple syrup)
1/2 tsp Cinnamon Dash Nutmeg or pumpkin pie spice
3-5 Stevia packets
1/2-1 cup Water
5-10 ice cubes
Optional: 1/2 tsp xanthan gum 3, ½ tsp butter extract

Directions:
1.   Add liquid first, then softer ingredients and harder items like ice or frozen fruit last.
2.   Blend on medium and increase to high for 1 minute. Repeat as necessary.

CHOCOLATE PEANUT BUTTER PROTEIN SMOOTHIE

Ingredients
1 large banana, peeled, sliced, and frozen
3 tbsps unsweetened cocoa powder
6 oz Chobani 0% Greek Yogurt (or 2%, flavored or unflavored)
3/4 cup skim milk
1 tbsp honey, maple syrup, or agave
1 tbsp peanut butter

Directions:
1.   Add liquid first, then softer ingredients and harder items like ice or frozen fruit last.
2.   Blend on medium and increase to high for 1 minute. Repeat as necessary.

GREEN WARRIOR PROTEIN SMOOTHIE

Ingredients

1/2 cup fresh red grapefruit juice
1 cup destemmed dinosaur/lacinato kale
1 large sweet apple, cored and roughly chopped
1 cup chopped cucumber
heaping 1/2 cup chopped celery (1 medium. stalk)
3-4 tbsps hemp hearts
1/4 cup frozen mango
1/8 cup fresh mint leaves
1/2 tbsp virgin coconut oil (optional)
3-4 ice cubes
1/2-1 tbsp algae oil, optional

Directions:
1.   Add liquid first, then softer ingredients and harder items like ice or frozen fruit last.
2.   Blend on medium and increase to high for 1 minute. Repeat as necessary.

COCONUT ALMOND PROTEIN SHAKE

Ingredients
For the nuts:
3/4 cup raw almonds
1/4 cup unsweetened shredded dried coconut
2 cups warm water
For the shake:
2 cups cold water
1 teaspoon kosher or celtic sea salt
1 rounded scoop vanilla protein powder (with no added sugar)
2 teaspoons grated fresh ginger
1 teaspoon ground cinnamon
1 teaspoon vanilla extract
2 tbsps coconut butter or coconut oil
Honey, to taste (optional)

Directions:
1.   Add liquid first, then softer ingredients and harder items like ice or frozen fruit last.
2.   Blend on medium and increase to high for 1 minute. Repeat as necessary.

BLUEBERRY PINEAPPLE OATMEAL SMOOTHIE

Ingredients
1 cup fresh blueberries
1 banana
½ pineapple, chopped into chunks
10 ice cubes
½ cup almond milk
½ cup of rolled oats
1 scoop of vanilla protein powder
½ cup of Greek yogurt
Directions:
1.   Add liquid first, then softer ingredients and harder items like ice or frozen fruit last.
2.   Blend on medium and increase to high for 1 minute. Repeat as necessary.

DARK CHOCOLATE PEPPERMINT PROTEIN SHAKE

Ingredients
1 large banana, frozen
2-3 large ice cubes
1 cup non dairy milk of choice
1 scoop Chocolate Protein Powder
2 tbsps cocoa powder
Pinch of sea salt
1/4 tsp pure peppermint extract
optional add In: 1 tbsp dark/vegan chocolate chips
optional toppings: homemade whipping cream, vegan whipped topping, or Greek yogurt
Directions:
1.   Add liquid first, then softer ingredients and harder items like ice or frozen fruit last.
2.   Blend on medium and increase to high for 1 minute. Repeat as necessary.

CHERRY ALMOND SMOOTHIE

Ingredients
1 cup of fresh or frozen pitted cherries

1 cup of almond or regular milk
2 tbsps of almond butter
3-4 ice cubes
1 scoop vanilla protein powder
Directions:
1.   Add liquid first, then softer ingredients and harder items like ice or frozen fruit last.
2.   Blend on medium and increase to high for 1 minute. Repeat as necessary.

CHOCOLATE ESPRESSO PROTEIN SMOOTHIE

Ingredients
1 banana, chunked and frozen
1 scoop chocolate protein powder
1 tsp instant coffee grounds {or ½ cup brewed coffee, chilled}
1 tsp unsweetened cocoa powder
1 tsp coconut palm sugar {optional}
1 cup coconut milk {or other milk}
½ cup ice {optional}
Directions:
1.   Add liquid first, then softer ingredients and harder items like ice or frozen fruit last.
2.   Blend on medium and increase to high for 1 minute. Repeat as necessary.

ROASTED STRAWBERRY PROTEIN SMOOTHIE

Ingredients
1-1/2 cups fresh strawberries, quartered
1/2 tbsp raw sugar
1/3 cup reduced fat cottage cheese
1/2 cup fat free milk
1 cup crushed ice
1 tsp chia seeds
6 to 8 drops liquid stevia (optional)
Directions:
1.   Add liquid first, then softer ingredients and harder items like ice or frozen fruit last.

2.   Blend on medium and increase to high for 1 minute. Repeat as necessary.

GREEN VANILLA ALMOND POST-WORKOUT SHAKE

Ingredients
1 cup unsweetened coconut milk
2 cups baby spinach
1 frozen banana
2 tbsps almond butter
2 teaspoons organic vanilla extract
1/4 cup (1 scoop) protein powder
1 cup ice
Directions:
1.   Add liquid first, then softer ingredients and harder items like ice or frozen fruit last.
2.   Blend on medium and increase to high for 1 minute. Repeat as necessary.

STRAWBERRY ALMOND PROTEIN DREAM SMOOTHIE

Ingredients
1 cup frozen organic strawberries
2 dates
1/2 cup almonds, soaked overnight
1/2 cup filtered water
Directions:
1.   Add liquid first, then softer ingredients and harder items like ice or frozen fruit last.
2.   Blend on medium and increase to high for 1 minute. Repeat as necessary.

ORANGE MANGO RECOVERY SMOOTHIE

Ingredients
1½ cups unsweetened almond milk
1 scoop vanilla vegan protein powder
1 cup frozen mango chunks
1 navel orange
2 tbsp cashews
1 tsp cinnamon
½ tsp turmeric
5 g fermented l-glutamine (optional)

Directions:
1.   Add liquid first, then softer ingredients and harder items like ice or frozen fruit last.
2.   Blend on medium and increase to high for 1 minute. Repeat as necessary.

THE PEANUT BUTTER POWER PROTEIN SHAKE

Ingredients
1 Scoop Chocolate Whey

2 tbsp. Natural Peanut butter
1/2 Banana
1 cup Skim Milk
1/4 cup Quaker Oats
2 ice cubes
Pinch of Salt
Directions:
1.   Add liquid first, then softer ingredients and harder items like ice or frozen fruit last.
2.   Blend on medium and increase to high for 1 minute. Repeat as necessary.

WINTER MINT CHOCOLATE PROTEIN SHAKE

Ingredients
1 Scoop Chocolate or Chocolate Mint Whey Protein Powder
1 cup almond Milk
1/2 cup No Sugar Added Mint Chocolate Chip Ice Cream
Optional, 1 Drop Peppermint Extract
Directions:
1.   Add liquid first, then softer ingredients and harder items like ice or frozen fruit last.
2.   Blend on medium and increase to high for 1 minute. Repeat as necessary.

CHERRY GINGER LIME SMOOTHIE

Ingredients
2 cups cherries, fresh or frozen

1 cup blueberries, fresh or frozen
1 whole lime, peeled
⅔ cup plain Greek yogurt
2 scoops protein powder
½ green apple
2 inch piece ginger root, thinly sliced
2 tbsps tart cherry juice
2 tbsps flax seed
1 cup water
ice to taste
Directions:
1.   Add liquid first, then softer ingredients and harder items like ice or frozen fruit last.
2.   Blend on medium and increase to high for 1 minute. Repeat as necessary.

20 WEIGHT-LOSS RECIPES

FAT BURNING GREEN TEA AND VEGETABLE SMOOTHIE

Ingredients
3 Broccoli Florets
2 Cauliflower Florets
2 Pineapple Spears
Green tea (ready-to-go)
Directions:
1.   Add liquid first, then softer ingredients and harder items like ice or frozen fruit last.
2.   Blend on medium and increase to high for 1 minute. Repeat as necessary.

CRISP APPLE SMOOTHIE

Ingredients
1 scoop protein powder
1 cup water
1 apple, cored, seeded and quartered
1 medium orange, peeled and quartered
1 banana, sliced
2 handfuls spinach
1 medium carrot, peeled and sliced
Directions:
1.   Add liquid first, then softer ingredients and harder items like ice or frozen fruit last.
(It helps a lot to blend fruits with liquid first before adding other ingredients. Check beginning of each section for special instructions)
2.   Blend on medium and increase to high for 1 minute. Repeat as necessary.

4 INGREDIENT GREEN SMOOTHIE

Ingredients
2 cups raw spinach
2 frozen medium bananas
1 cup fresh, whole strawberries
1 cup unsweetened vanilla almond milk
Directions:
1.   Add liquid first, then softer ingredients and harder items like ice or frozen fruit last.
(It helps a lot to blend fruits with liquid first before adding other ingredients. Check beginning of each section for special instructions)
2.   Blend on medium and increase to high for 1 minute. Repeat as necessary.

5 INGREDIENT CREAMY BANANA GREEN SMOOTHIE

Ingredients
1 banana
1 avocado
2 cups(450g) spinach
1 green apple
1 cup (240 g) Greek yogurt
Directions:
1.   Add liquid first, then softer ingredients and harder items like ice or frozen fruit last.
(It helps a lot to blend fruits with liquid first before adding other ingredients. Check beginning of each section for special instructions)
2.   Blend on medium and increase to high for 1 minute. Repeat as necessary.

GREEN SUPERFOOD SMOOTHIE

Ingredients
½ cup water
1½ cups freshly squeezed grapefruit juice
2 cups spinach
1 tsp spirulina
2 kiwis
1 avocado
½ cup frozen mango chunks
Directions:

1.   Add liquid first, then softer ingredients and harder items like ice or frozen fruit last.
(It helps a lot to blend fruits with liquid first before adding other ingredients. Check beginning of each section for special instructions)
2.   Blend on medium and increase to high for 1 minute. Repeat as necessary.

TROPICAL GREENS SMOOTHIE

Ingredients
1 1/2 cups fresh watermelon chunks
Juice of one lime
1 large handful of fresh baby spinach
2 sprigs of fresh curly parsley
2 sprigs of fresh mint
1/2 cup frozen strawberries
1 cup frozen pineapple tidbits
1/2 cup frozen mango chunks
1/2 cup green tea or coconut water
Directions:
1.   Add liquid first, then softer ingredients and harder items like ice or frozen fruit last.
(It helps a lot to blend fruits with liquid first before adding other ingredients. Check beginning of each section for special instructions)
2.   Blend on medium and increase to high for 1 minute. Repeat as necessary.

BLUEBERRY PINEAPPLE GREEN DETOX SMOOTHIE

Ingredients
1 cup baby spinach or baby kale
1 cup fresh really ripe pineapple, cored and cut into chunks
½ cup plain Greek yogurt non-fat
2 teaspoons of ground cinnamon
dash of turmeric
1-2 teaspoons of chia seeds, flaxseed
1 small knob the size of a quarter of fresh ginger root

juice from ½ lemon
½ cup water, milk or juice
2 cups frozen blueberries
Directions:
1.   Add liquid first, then softer ingredients and harder items like ice or frozen fruit last.
(It helps a lot to blend fruits with liquid first before adding other ingredients. Check beginning of each section for special instructions)
2.   Blend on medium and increase to high for 1 minute. Repeat as necessary.

RASPBERRY MANGO CHIA SEED SMOOTHIE

Ingredients
1 cup apple juice frozen concentrate
1. 5 cups frozen raspberries
1.5 cup frozen mango chunks
2 cups spinach
2 Tbs Chia seeds
Water
Directions:
1.   Add liquid first, then softer ingredients and harder items like ice or frozen fruit last.
(It helps a lot to blend fruits with liquid first before adding other ingredients. Check beginning of each section for special instructions)
2.   Blend on medium and increase to high for 1 minute. Repeat as necessary.

TROPICAL GREEN SMOOTHIE
Ingredients
1 medium mango, peeled and cubed
2 cups watermelon, cubed
1 large kale leaf or spinach
½ cup freshly squeezed orange juice
1 cup coconut water
1/4 teaspoon freshly ground black pepper
a few mint leaves
Directions:

1.   Add liquid first, then softer ingredients and harder items like ice or frozen fruit last.
(It helps a lot to blend fruits with liquid first before adding other ingredients. Check beginning of each section for special instructions)
2.   Blend on medium and increase to high for 1 minute. Repeat as necessary.

FRUITY GREEN SMOOTHIE

Ingredients
½ large bunch of kale, stems removed
2 cups pineapple rings
1 mango
1 ripe banana (optional)
1-2 cups water
coconut water
Directions:
1.   Add liquid first, then softer ingredients and harder items like ice or frozen fruit last.
(It helps a lot to blend fruits with liquid first before adding other ingredients. Check beginning of each section for special instructions)
2.   Blend on medium and increase to high for 1 minute. Repeat as necessary.

RAINBOW SMOOTHIE

Ingredients
Layer 1 Banana/almond:
130g crushed ice2 small bananas (about 80g each with skin removed)
10 almonds
50ml semi skimmed milk
Layer 2 Kale/date:
50g crushed ice
2 medjool dates, stones removed and roughly chopped
75g kale
Layer 3 blueberry
80g crushed ice
70g blueberries
50ml water

Layer 4 Strawberry/milk
80g crushed ice
80g strawberries, green bits cut off
50ml semi skimmed milk
Directions:
1.   Add liquid first, then softer ingredients and harder items like ice or frozen fruit last.
(It helps a lot to blend fruits with liquid first before adding other ingredients. Check beginning of each section for special instructions)
2.   Blend on medium and increase to high for 1 minute. Repeat as necessary.

VERY CHERRY GREEN SMOOTHIE

Ingredients
1 cup frozen cherries
1/2 cup frozen mango chunks
2 cups organic spinach
<u>100% baby kale</u>
1 banana
2 cups pomegranate-blueberry juice
Directions:
1.   Add liquid first, then softer ingredients and harder items like ice or frozen fruit last.
(It helps a lot to blend fruits with liquid first before adding other ingredients. Check beginning of each section for special instructions)
2.   Blend on medium and increase to high for 1 minute. Repeat as necessary.

CREAMY AVOCADO KALE SMOOTHIE

Ingredients
½ an Avocado
½ cup Kale
1 TBSP cacao Nibs
½ cup Greek Yogurt
½ cup Vanilla almond Milk
½ cup Frozen Mango
2 tsp Honey

Directions:
1.   Add liquid first, then softer ingredients and harder items like ice or frozen fruit last.
(It helps a lot to blend fruits with liquid first before adding other ingredients. Check beginning of each section for special instructions)
2.   Blend on medium and increase to high for 1 minute. Repeat as necessary.

BERRIES AND OATS SMOOTHIE

Ingredients
12 ounces coconut water
2 small oranges (or 1 large)
1 cup blueberries
2 cups strawberries
2 cups spinach
1 medium banana
2 cups ice (less if using frozen fruit)
1/2 cup rolled oats
Directions:
1.   Add liquid first, then softer ingredients and harder items like ice or frozen fruit last.
(It helps a lot to blend fruits with liquid first before adding other ingredients. Check beginning of each section for special instructions)
2.   Blend on medium and increase to high for 1 minute. Repeat as necessary.

GREEN BLUEBERRY BANANA SMOOTHIE

Ingredients
1 cup skim milk (or milk of choice)
1/3 cup plain nonfat Greek yogurt
1 frozen banana
3/4 cup frozen blueberries
1 cup baby spinach
1 T. flaxseed meal
4 t. maple syrup or honey
1/2 t. vanilla extract

1 T. unsweetened shredded coconut (optional)
Directions:
1.   Add liquid first, then softer ingredients and harder items like ice or frozen fruit last.
(It helps a lot to blend fruits with liquid first before adding other ingredients. Check beginning of each section for special instructions)
2.   Blend on medium and increase to high for 1 minute. Repeat as necessary.

LULU'S GREEN SMOOTHIE

Ingredients
A big fistful of baby spinach or baby kale (roughly 1 cup packed)
1 ripe banana, cold
1/4 avocado, cold
2 cups original or vanilla soymilk
Optional: fresh mint leaves or a dash cinnamon
2-3 ice cubes
Directions:
1.   Add liquid first, then softer ingredients and harder items like ice or frozen fruit last.
(It helps a lot to blend fruits with liquid first before adding other ingredients. Check beginning of each section for special instructions)
2.   Blend on medium and increase to high for 1 minute. Repeat as necessary.

BLUEBERRY PEACH KALE CHIA SMOOTHIE

Ingredients
2 cups coconut milk or almond milk
2 cups blueberries (fresh or frozen)
1 cup peaches (fresh or frozen)
1 cup kale
1 small banana (fresh or frozen)
1 tbsp Chia seeds
1 tbsp honey
1 1/2 cups ice (less if using frozen fruit)

Directions:
1.   Add liquid first, then softer ingredients and harder items like ice or frozen fruit last.
(It helps a lot to blend fruits with liquid first before adding other ingredients. Check beginning of each section for special instructions)
2.   Blend on medium and increase to high for 1 minute. Repeat as necessary.

GREEN SMOOTHIE BOWL

Ingredients
1 handful of baby spinach leaves
1 handful of baby kale leaves
2 medium sized carrots
1 large very ripe banana
1 cup of blueberries
2 tbsps of hemp protein powder
1/3 cup of unsweetened almond milk
1 tbsp of almond butter
Directions:
1.   Add liquid first, then softer ingredients and harder items like ice or frozen fruit last.
(It helps a lot to blend fruits with liquid first before adding other ingredients. Check beginning of each section for special instructions)
2.   Blend on medium and increase to high for 1 minute. Repeat as necessary.

GRAPE MANGO KALE SMOOTHIE

Ingredients
8 ounces coconut water
1/2 cup red grapes
1/2 cup watermelon
1 cup mango, fresh or frozen
1 cup kale
1 carrot, cut into chunks
juice of 1/2 lemon
1 date
1 1/2 cups of ice
Directions:

1.   Add liquid first, then softer ingredients and harder items like ice or frozen fruit last.
(It helps a lot to blend fruits with liquid first before adding other ingredients. Check beginning of each section for special instructions)
2.   Blend on medium and increase to high for 1 minute. Repeat as necessary.

GREEN GOODNESS IN A GLASS

Ingredients
1 Green Apple
2 Beetroot Leaves
2-3 Kale Leaves
1/2 Small Avocado
Ice cubes
Lots of Cinnamon
5 cm Piece of Cucumber
Milk of choice (rice, almond, soy, coconut water or just water.)
Directions:
1.   Add liquid first, then softer ingredients and harder items like ice or frozen fruit last.
(It helps a lot to blend fruits with liquid first before adding other ingredients. Check beginning of each section for special instructions)
2.   Blend on medium and increase to high for 1 minute. Repeat as necessary.

10 ANTI-AGING RECIPES

BLUEBERRY PEACH ANTI AGING SMOOTHIE

Ingredients
½ cup fresh or frozen blueberries
1½ cup fresh sliced peach, with peel or frozen peaches, pits removed
About ¾ cup unsweetened vanilla almond milk, to the fill line

Directions:
1. Add liquid first, then softer ingredients and harder items like ice or frozen fruit last.
(It helps a lot to blend fruits with liquid first before adding other ingredients. Check beginning of each section for special instructions)
2. Blend on medium and increase to high for 1 minute. Repeat as necessary.

ANTI-AGING TURMERIC SMOOTHIE

Ingredients
1 cup coconut milk
1/2 cup frozen pineapple or mango chunks
1 fresh banana
1 tbsp coconut oil
1 teaspoon turmeric
1/2 teaspoon cinnamon
1/2 teaspoon ginger
1/2 avocado

Directions:
1. Add liquid first, then softer ingredients and harder items like ice or frozen fruit last.
(It helps a lot to blend fruits with liquid first before adding other ingredients. Check beginning of each section for special instructions)
2. Blend on medium and increase to high for 1 minute. Repeat as necessary.

CHOCOLATE BERRY ALMOND BLAST

Ingredients
1 cup Spinach
1 tbsp cacao Nibs
1 tbsp almond butter
½ cup Cherries, frozen
½ cup Mixed Berries
1 Splash Vanilla
½ teaspoon Ceylon Cinnamon
1 ½ cups almond Milk

Directions:
1. Add liquid first, then softer ingredients and harder items like ice or frozen fruit last.
(It helps a lot to blend fruits with liquid first before adding other ingredients. Check beginning of each section for special instructions)
2. Blend on medium and increase to high for 1 minute. Repeat as necessary.

BLUEBERRY DETOX SMOOTHIE

Ingredients
1 cup wild frozen blueberries, or just frozen blueberries
1 cup cubed raw red beets, peeled
1 cup cubed watermelon
1 cup coconut water
1 teaspoon chia seeds (optional)
1 handful of basil leaves (or mint)

Directions:
1. Add liquid first, then softer ingredients and harder items like ice or frozen fruit last.
(It helps a lot to blend fruits with liquid first before adding other ingredients. Check beginning of each section for special instructions)
2. Blend on medium and increase to high for 1 minute. Repeat as necessary.

ALKALINE CLEANSING SMOOTHIE

Ingredients
1 rib of celery
1/4 cucumber
1 handful of cilantro
1 handful of parsley
1/2 lemon, peeled
A slice of ginger
Directions:
1.   Add liquid first, then softer ingredients and harder items like ice or frozen fruit last.
(It helps a lot to blend fruits with liquid first before adding other ingredients. Check beginning of each section for special instructions)
2.   Blend on medium and increase to high for 1 minute. Repeat as necessary.

TANGERINE TURMERIC ANTIOXIDANT SMOOTHIE

Ingredients
2 tangerines, peeled
1 large organic carrot, chopped
½ avocado
1 cup coconut milk
1 teaspoon turmeric
1 teaspoon Dole milled chia seeds
5-6 ice cubes
Directions:
1.   Add liquid first, then softer ingredients and harder items like ice or frozen fruit last.
(It helps a lot to blend fruits with liquid first before adding other ingredients. Check beginning of each section for special instructions)
2.   Blend on medium and increase to high for 1 minute. Repeat as necessary.

RED GRAPE, PLUM, AND RASPBERRY ANTIOXIDANT SMOOTHIE

Ingredients
1 cup red seedless grapes
2 handfuls spinach
3 red plums, pits removed
½ cup raspberries
Directions:
1.   Add liquid first, then softer ingredients and harder items like ice or frozen fruit last.
2.   (It helps a lot to blend fruits with liquid first before adding other ingredients. Check beginning of each section for special instructions)
3.   Blend on medium and increase to high for 1 minute. Repeat as necessary.

AN ANTI-AGING SMOOTHIE

Ingredients
1 1/2 cup Kale Cut Up
2 Celery Sticks
1 Juice Whole Lemon
1 Medium Apple (Cored)
1 handful Parsley
1 1/2 cup coconut Water
Directions:
1.   Add liquid first, then softer ingredients and harder items like ice or frozen fruit last.
(It helps a lot to blend fruits with liquid first before adding other ingredients. Check beginning of each section for special instructions)
2.   Blend on medium and increase to high for 1 minute. Repeat as necessary.

GO, GO, GOJI BLAST

Ingredients
1 Banana
1 tbsp _cacao
¼ cup Goji Berries
½ cup Grapes
½ cup Blueberries
1 tbsp Honey
3 _ice cubes
To Max Line Water

Directions:
1.   Add liquid first, then softer ingredients and harder items like ice or frozen fruit last.
(It helps a lot to blend fruits with liquid first before adding other ingredients. Check beginning of each section for special instructions)
2.   Blend on medium and increase to high for 1 minute. Repeat as necessary.

WATERMELON SMOOTHIE

Ingredients
1½ cups Watermelon (seedless or remove seeds)
1 frozen banana
1 apple, peeled and cored
¾ cup fat free Thick Greek Yogurt
Agave or honey
Directions:
1.   Add liquid first, then softer ingredients and harder items like ice or frozen fruit last.
(It helps a lot to blend fruits with liquid first before adding other ingredients. Check beginning of each section for special instructions)
2.   Blend on medium and increase to high for 1 minute. Repeat as necessary.

10 DETOXIFICATION RECIPES

DETOX SMOOTHIE

Ingredients
1 frozen sliced very ripe banana, previously peeled & sliced
1/4 cup almond milk
1 and 1/4 cups chopped pineapple
1 peach, peeled and sliced
1/2 cup Greek yogurt
1 - 2 cups fresh spinach
Juice + zest of 1 lime, optional (provides great flavor)
Directions:
1.   Add liquid first, then softer ingredients and harder items like ice or frozen fruit last.
(It helps a lot to blend fruits with liquid first before adding other ingredients. Check beginning of each section for special instructions)
2.   Blend on medium and increase to high for 1 minute. Repeat as necessary.

CITRUS & GREEN TEA DETOX SMOOTHIE

Ingredients
1 navel orange
1 grapefruit
the juice of half a lemon
1/2 cup of unsweetened green tea, chilled
1/2 cup of nonfat Greek yogurt
1/2 a frozen banana
1 cup of ice
1/2 tbsp honey
optional garnishes: orange/grapefruit/lemon zest on top
Directions:
1.   Add liquid first, then softer ingredients and harder items like ice or frozen fruit last.
(It helps a lot to blend fruits with liquid first before adding other ingredients. Check beginning of each section for special instructions)
2.   Blend on medium and increase to high for 1 minute. Repeat as necessary.

DETOX BLUEBERRY FRUIT SMOOTHIE

Ingredients
½ cup frozen blueberries
¼ cup unsweetened cranberry juice
1-2 bananas
Directions:
1.   Add liquid first, then softer ingredients and harder items like ice or frozen fruit last.
(It helps a lot to blend fruits with liquid first before adding other ingredients. Check beginning of each section for special instructions)
2.   Blend on medium and increase to high for 1 minute. Repeat as necessary.

LEMON GINGER DETOX DRINK

Ingredients
1 12-ounce glass water, at room temperature
Juice of 1/2 lemon
1/2 inch knob of ginger root
Directions:
1.   Add liquid first, then softer ingredients and harder items like ice or frozen fruit last.
(It helps a lot to blend fruits with liquid first before adding other ingredients. Check beginning of each section for special instructions)
2.   Blend on medium and increase to high for 1 minute. Repeat as necessary.

DETOX BEET AND CARROT SMOOTHIE

Ingredients

1 carrot, peeled, sliced
1 beet, peeled, sliced
½ cup red grapes
1 clementine, peeled
1 slice of ginger, peeled, about the size of a quarter
½ cup green tea
Directions:
1.   Add liquid first, then softer ingredients and harder items like ice or frozen fruit last.
(It helps a lot to blend fruits with liquid first before adding other ingredients. Check beginning of each section for special instructions)
2.   Blend on medium and increase to high for 1 minute. Repeat as necessary.v

GRAPEFRUIT-CADO SUNRISE SMOOTHIE

Ingredients
1/2 avocado
1/2 cup fresh squeezed orange juice
1 cup fresh squeezed grapefruit juice
1 cup DOLE frozen strawberries
3/4 cup DOLE banana (use frozen banana slices for thicker smoothie)
1/4 cup ice
optional: 1 tsp maple syrup
Directions:
1.   Add liquid first, then softer ingredients and harder items like ice or frozen fruit last.
(It helps a lot to blend fruits with liquid first before adding other ingredients. Check beginning of each section for special instructions)
2.   Blend on medium and increase to high for 1 minute. Repeat as necessary.

NATURAL DAILY DETOX REMEDY DRINK

Ingredients
16-25 oz Cold Water
1-2 tbsp Apple Cider Vinegar

1 Full Lemon
Ice
Optional:
Cinnamon
Stevia
Directions:
1.   Add liquid first, then softer ingredients and harder items like ice or frozen fruit last.
(It helps a lot to blend fruits with liquid first before adding other ingredients. Check beginning of each section for special instructions)
2.   Blend on medium and increase to high for 1 minute. Repeat as necessary.

MATCHA MANGO PINEAPPLE SMOOTHIE

Ingredients
1.25 tsp matcha green tea
1 scoop protein powder
some honey
1 c frozen mango chunks
1 tbsp pineapple juice
1 c pineapple
1/2 to 1 c water
Directions:
1.   Add liquid first, then softer ingredients and harder items like ice or frozen fruit last.
(It helps a lot to blend fruits with liquid first before adding other ingredients. Check beginning of each section for special instructions)
2.   Blend on medium and increase to high for 1 minute. Repeat as necessary.

SPRING CLEANING DETOX

Ingredients
1 teaspoon of whole flax seeds.
1 red apple, peeled and sliced.
8 snack-sized peeled carrots (or 2 normal carrots, peeled and chopped).
1/4 inch nub of fresh ginger root, skin removed. (should be moist)

1 cup of lukewarm water.
Directions:
1.   Add liquid first, then softer ingredients and harder items like ice or frozen fruit last.
(It helps a lot to blend fruits with liquid first before adding other ingredients. Check beginning of each section for special instructions)
2.   Blend on medium and increase to high for 1 minute. Repeat as necessary.

CRANBERRY BLISS DETOX SMOOTHIE

Ingredients
2 apples, sliced, peel left on
2 pears, sliced, peel left on
1 lemon, peeled, cut in quarters, seeds removed
1 cup fresh cranberries
2 cups of filtered water
Sweetener of choice
4-6 Ice cubes
1 tbsp turmeric
2 teaspoons pumpkin pie spice blend (optional) OR 2 teaspoons of cinnamon or 1 teaspoon of nutmeg
Directions:
1.   Add liquid first, then softer ingredients and harder items like ice or frozen fruit last.
(It helps a lot to blend fruits with liquid first before adding other ingredients. Check beginning of each section for special instructions)
2.   Blend on medium and increase to high for 1 minute. Repeat as necessary.

F.10 ENERGY BOOSTING RECIPES

AFTERNOON ENERGY SMOOTHIE

Ingredients
2 medium bananas (Peeled)
3 whole Medjool dates (Pits removed)
1 cup unsweetened almond milk
1 TBSP hulled hemp seeds
1/2 cup ice (optional)
Directions:
1.   Add liquid first, then softer ingredients and harder items like ice or frozen fruit last.
(It helps a lot to blend fruits with liquid first before adding other ingredients. Check beginning of each section for special instructions)
2.   Blend on medium and increase to high for 1 minute. Repeat as necessary.

ENERGY BOOST FRUIT SMOOTHIE

Ingredients
1 cup of pineapple, peeled and chopped
1 medium orange, peeled
1 cup raspberries
1 medium banana, peeled
1 cup almond milk
1 cup crushed ice
Directions:
1.   Add liquid first, then softer ingredients and harder items like ice or frozen fruit last.
(It helps a lot to blend fruits with liquid first before adding other ingredients. Check beginning of each section for special instructions)
2.   Blend on medium and increase to high for 1 minute. Repeat as necessary.

BLUEBERRY ALMOND BUTTER SMOOTHIES

Ingredients
1 banana, peeled
1 cup frozen blueberries
1/2 cup almond butter
1/2 cup plain yogurt
3/4 cup almond milk
3 dates, pitted and quartered
1 cup ice, or as needed
Directions:
1.   Add liquid first, then softer ingredients and harder items like ice or frozen fruit last.
(It helps a lot to blend fruits with liquid first before adding other ingredients. Check beginning of each section for special instructions)
2.   Blend on medium and increase to high for 1 minute. Repeat as necessary.

FRUIT AND VEGGIE SMOOTHIE

Ingredients
2 carrots
3 tomatoes
2 apples
1 cucumber
3 slices of pineapple
4 beets
chunk of ginger
lemon
2 bell peppers
Directions:
1.   Add liquid first, then softer ingredients and harder items like ice or frozen fruit last.
(It helps a lot to blend fruits with liquid first before adding other ingredients. Check beginning of each section for special instructions)
2.   Blend on medium and increase to high for 1 minute. Repeat as necessary.

MANGO-STRAWBERRY WATERMELON SMOOTHIE

Ingredients
1 peeled and sliced Mango
6-10 Strawberries depending on tartness
3-4 cups chopped Watermelon
1 tbsp Honey (optional)
Directions:
1.   Add liquid first, then softer ingredients and harder items like ice or frozen fruit last.
(It helps a lot to blend fruits with liquid first before adding other ingredients. Check beginning of each section for special instructions)
2.   Blend on medium and increase to high for 1 minute. Repeat as necessary.

RAW MANGO LASSI

Ingredients
2 Large fresh ripe organic Mangoes
1 banana
½ cup of organic hemp hearts (can substitute coconut meat instead)
1 teaspoon of chai spice.
1 cup of either almond milk, coconut milk, or coconut water.
Directions:
1.   Add liquid first, then softer ingredients and harder items like ice or frozen fruit last.
(It helps a lot to blend fruits with liquid first before adding other ingredients. Check beginning of each section for special instructions)
2.   Blend on medium and increase to high for 1 minute. Repeat as necessary.

DR. OZ'S ENERGY BOOST SMOOTHIE

Ingredients
2 tbsp. pure cocoa powder
2 tbsp creamy natural peanut butter

1 medium ripe banana
8 oz nonfat vanilla Greek yogurt
1/2 cup almond Milk
4 to 6 ice cubes
1/2 tsp cinnamon
Directions:
1.   Add liquid first, then softer ingredients and harder items like ice or frozen fruit last.
(It helps a lot to blend fruits with liquid first before adding other ingredients. Check beginning of each section for special instructions)
2.   Blend on medium and increase to high for 1 minute. Repeat as necessary.

LUSH CHERRY AND COCONUT SMOOTHIE

Ingredients
1/2 cup pitted cherries, frozen or fresh
1/4 cup (30 g / 1 oz / handful) frozen raspberries
Juice + flesh from 1 young coconut
2 scoops whey protein
1 teaspoon chia seed
Directions:
1.   Add liquid first, then softer ingredients and harder items like ice or frozen fruit last.
(It helps a lot to blend fruits with liquid first before adding other ingredients. Check beginning of each section for special instructions)
2.   Blend on medium and increase to high for 1 minute. Repeat as necessary.

KIWI & GREEN TEA SMOOTHIE

Ingredients
Makes 4 cups (500 ml)
2 cups (500 ml) maché salad (also called lamb's lettuce, valerian, corn salad)
2 kiwi
1 1/2 banana, frozen

1 cup pineapple (250 ml)
1 cup green tea, cold (250 ml)
Directions:
1.   Add liquid first, then softer ingredients and harder items like ice or frozen fruit last.
(It helps a lot to blend fruits with liquid first before adding other ingredients. Check beginning of each section for special instructions)
2.   Blend on medium and increase to high for 1 minute. Repeat as necessary.

PEANUT BUTTER AND BANANA OATMEAL SMOOTHIE

Ingredients
1 banana
1 cup plain yogurt
2 tbsp. peanut butter
1/2 cup milk
1/4 cup quick-cooking oats and a squirt of honey to taste.
Directions:
1.   Add liquid first, then softer ingredients and harder items like ice or frozen fruit last.
(It helps a lot to blend fruits with liquid first before adding other ingredients. Check beginning of each section for special instructions)
2.   Blend on medium and increase to high for 1 minute. Repeat as necessary.

10 HIGH-CALORIE RECIPES (TO STAY FULL LONGER)

STRAWBERRY MANGO AND ALMOND SMOOTHIE

Ingredients
1 cup strawberries (fresh or frozen)
½ cup mango
3-4 almonds (soaked overnight)
coconut milk to the fill line
1 teaspoon honey
Directions:
1.   Add liquid first, then softer ingredients and harder items like ice or frozen fruit last.
(It helps a lot to blend fruits with liquid first before adding other ingredients. Check beginning of each section for special instructions)
2.   Blend on medium and increase to high for 1 minute. Repeat as necessary.

RASPBERRY CHEESECAKE SMOOTHIE

Ingredients
½ cup skim milk
½ cup nonfat cottage cheese
2 tbsps honey
½ tsp vanilla extract
1 cup raspberries
Directions:
1. Add liquid first, then softer ingredients and harder items like ice or frozen fruit last.
(It helps a lot to blend fruits with liquid first before adding other ingredients. Check beginning of each section for special instructions)
2. Blend on medium and increase to high for 1 minute. Repeat as necessary.

SWEET POTATO AND BANANA PIE SMOOTHIE

Ingredients
2 cups *Water*
1 cup of Sweet potato (cooked)
4 *Bananas* (4 cups)
½ cup *Raisins* / Sultanas (or any dried fruit)
¼ cup *Pecans* (Or any other nuts or plain seeds)
1 teaspoon *Cinnamon*
¼ cup Dried *coconut* (Or any other type of coconut)
Directions:
1. Add liquid first, then softer ingredients and harder items like ice or frozen fruit last.
(It helps a lot to blend fruits with liquid first before adding other ingredients. Check beginning of each section for special instructions)
2. Blend on medium and increase to high for 1 minute. Repeat as necessary.

TROPICAL PROTEIN SHAKE SMOOTHIE

Ingredients
1 cup fresh pineapple
1 medium kiwi, skin intact
2 T unsweetened coconut
6 almonds
1 cup vanilla Greek yogurt
coconut milk to the fill line
Directions:
1. Add liquid first, then softer ingredients and harder items like ice or frozen fruit last.
(It helps a lot to blend fruits with liquid first before adding other ingredients. Check beginning of each section for special instructions)
2. Blend on medium and increase to high for 1 minute. Repeat as necessary.

MORNING ENERGY BLAST

Ingredients
1 Banana
2 tbsps Peanut butter
½ cup Greek Yogurt
2 tbsps _cacao
1 Dash Cinnamon
 ice cubes
To Max Line Water
Directions:
 1. Add liquid first, then softer
ingredients and harder items like ice or
frozen fruit last.
 (It helps a lot to blend fruits with liquid
first before adding other ingredients.
Check beginning of each section for
special instructions)
 2. Blend on medium and increase to
high for 1 minute. Repeat as necessary.

ALMOND BUTTER ME UP!

Ingredients
1 Handful Spinach
½ Bananas
1 tbsp_almond_butter
1 Handful Mixed Berries
1 tbsp SuperFood Protein Boost
To Max Line coconut Water
Directions:
 1. Add liquid first, then softer
ingredients and harder items like ice or
frozen fruit last.
 (It helps a lot to blend fruits with liquid
first before adding other ingredients.
Check beginning of each section for
special instructions)
 2. Blend on medium and increase to
high for 1 minute. Repeat as necessary.

ENERGY BLAST CITRUS GREEN SMOOTHIE

Ingredients
2 big handfuls of fresh spinach
2 large oranges (or 4 clementines)
1 large red grapefruit

1 1/2 cups of water, orange or
grapefruit juice.
1 tbsp of Chia Seeds
Directions:
 1. Add liquid first, then softer
ingredients and harder items like ice or
frozen fruit last.
 (It helps a lot to blend fruits with liquid
first before adding other ingredients.
Check beginning of each section for
special instructions)
 2. Blend on medium and increase to
high for 1 minute. Repeat as necessary.

PINEAPPLE GINGER ENERGY BLAST

Ingredients
1 cup Spinach
1 Small Banana
½ cup Greek Yogurt
1 tbsp Ginger
1 cup Pineapple
ice cubes
To Max Line Water
Directions:
 1. Add liquid first, then softer
ingredients and harder items like ice or
frozen fruit last.
 (It helps a lot to blend fruits with liquid
first before adding other ingredients.
Check beginning of each section for
special instructions)
 2. Blend on medium and increase to
high for 1 minute. Repeat as necessary.

CHOCOLATE-COVERED CHERRY SMOOTHIE

Ingredients
3/4 cup frozen dark sweet cherries
1 cup 35-calorie almond milk
1 scoop CytoSport 100% Whey Protein
1 tbsp unsweetened cocoa powder
1/3 cup baby carrots (optional)
For the topping
1/2 cup whipping cream

1 package Stevia
Directions:
 1. Add liquid first, then softer
ingredients and harder items like ice or
frozen fruit last.
 (It helps a lot to blend fruits with liquid
first before adding other ingredients.
Check beginning of each section for
special instructions)
 2. Blend on medium and increase to
high for 1 minute. Repeat as necessary.

ALMOND DELIGHT

Ingredients
1 cup Mixed Greens
½ cup Raspberries
½ cup Strawberries
½ cup Garbanzo Beans
1 tbsp almond_butter
1 scoop whey protein powder
½ teaspoon Cinnamon
To Max Line Water
Directions:
 1. Add liquid first, then softer
ingredients and harder items like ice or
frozen fruit last.
 (It helps a lot to blend fruits with liquid
first before adding other ingredients.
Check beginning of each section for
special instructions)
 2. Blend on medium and increase to
high for 1 minute. Repeat as necessary.

100 JUICE RECIPES

CARROT, PEAR, RASPBERRY, CUCUMBER JUICE

Ingredients
4 or 5 carrots
1 pear
12 ounces of organic raspberries
1 cucumber
Directions:
1. Add liquid first, then softer ingredients and harder items like ice or frozen fruit last.
(It helps a lot to blend fruits with liquid first before adding other ingredients. Check beginning of each section for special instructions)
2. Blend on medium and increase to high for 1 minute. Repeat as necessary.

PINKY PROMISE CARROT JUICE

Ingredients
3 organic carrots
1 apple
½ inch piece of ginger
a few sprigs of parsley
Directions:
1. Add liquid first, then softer ingredients and harder items like ice or frozen fruit last.
(It helps a lot to blend fruits with liquid first before adding other ingredients. Check beginning of each section for special instructions)
2. Blend on medium and increase to high for 1 minute. Repeat as necessary.

BEET GREEN, CARROT, APPLE, ORANGE JUICE

Ingredients
5 peeled carrots
1 bunch beet greens (about 5-6 large), can also use chard
2 small oranges, peeled and and cut into half through the equator, seeds removed
2 apples, cut into quarters, cores removed
Directions:
1. Add liquid first, then softer ingredients and harder items like ice or frozen fruit last.
(It helps a lot to blend fruits with liquid first before adding other ingredients. Check beginning of each section for special instructions)
2. Blend on medium and increase to high for 1 minute. Repeat as necessary.

THE ULTIMATE GREEN POWER JUICE

Ingredients
6 large Fuji or Gala apples, quartered
4 cups baby spinach leaves
1 bunch of parsley
2 inches fresh ginger, skin removed
1 lemon
Directions:
1. Add liquid first, then softer ingredients and harder items like ice or frozen fruit last.
(It helps a lot to blend fruits with liquid first before adding other ingredients. Check beginning of each section for special instructions)
2. Blend on medium and increase to high for 1 minute. Repeat as necessary.

LAUREN'S FAVORITE GREEN JUICE

Ingredients
2 cups baby spinach {packed full}
1/2 english cucumber, peeled
3 fuji apples
2 navel oranges
1 ruby red grapefruit
1 small lemon, peeled {optional}
Directions:

1. Add liquid first, then softer ingredients and harder items like ice or frozen fruit last.

(It helps a lot to blend fruits with liquid first before adding other ingredients. Check beginning of each section for special instructions)

2. Blend on medium and increase to high for 1 minute. Repeat as necessary.

V8 JUICE

Ingredients

1 tbsp extra virgin olive oil
5 medium-large tomatoes, chopped
½ onion, chopped
2 cloves garlic
1 beet, chopped
1 carrot, chopped
1 tbsp honey
1 dash tabasco sauce
1 dash worcestershire sauce
salt & pepper
2 small cucumbers, chopped
¼ cup fresh parsley

Directions:

1. Add liquid first, then softer ingredients and harder items like ice or frozen fruit last.

(It helps a lot to blend fruits with liquid first before adding other ingredients. Check beginning of each section for special instructions)

2. Blend on medium and increase to high for 1 minute. Repeat as necessary.

GRAPEFRUIT VEGGIE LIME JUICE

Ingredients

1 pink grapefruit, peeled, sliced
2 celery stalks, chopped
1 red pepper, cored, stem removed
1/2 lime, skin removed

Directions:

1. Add liquid first, then softer ingredients and harder items like ice or frozen fruit last.

(It helps a lot to blend fruits with liquid first before adding other ingredients. Check beginning of each section for special instructions)

2. Blend on medium and increase to high for 1 minute. Repeat as necessary.

GRAPEFRUIT MINT JUICE

Ingredients

2 grapefruits, peeled and sectioned to fit into the juicer
8-10 leaves of fresh mint

Directions:

1. Add liquid first, then softer ingredients and harder items like ice or frozen fruit last.

(It helps a lot to blend fruits with liquid first before adding other ingredients. Check beginning of each section for special instructions)

2. Blend on medium and increase to high for 1 minute. Repeat as necessary.

CARROT, ORANGE, AND GINGER JUICE WITHOUT JUICER

Ingredients

6 carrots, peeled and cut into large chunks
1 orange, peeled and cut into large chunks
1/2-inch piece of fresh ginger root, peeling removed
1 cup water
ice

Directions:

1. Add liquid first, then softer ingredients and harder items like ice or frozen fruit last.

(It helps a lot to blend fruits with liquid first before adding other ingredients.

Check beginning of each section for special instructions)

2. Blend on medium and increase to high for 1 minute. Repeat as necessary.

GREEN JUICE WITHOUT A JUICER

Ingredients
3 handfuls of kale (or about 3 loosely packed cups)
1 whole apple, cored and cut into large chunks
1 stalk of celery, cut into large chunks
1/2 English cucumber, cut into large chunks
juice from 1/2 a lime
1 handful of parsley or about 1 cup loosely packed
1 cup water
Ice

Directions:
1. Add liquid first, then softer ingredients and harder items like ice or frozen fruit last.

(It helps a lot to blend fruits with liquid first before adding other ingredients. Check beginning of each section for special instructions)

2. Blend on medium and increase to high for 1 minute. Repeat as necessary.

GREEN JUICE IN A BLENDER

Ingredients
1 1/2 cups water
2 cups kale
2 green apples, cored
1/2 cup parsley leaves
1 medium cucumber, quartered
2 celery stalks, roughly chopped
1 (1-inch) piece of ginger, peeled
2 tbsps lemon juice

Directions:
1. Add liquid first, then softer ingredients and harder items like ice or frozen fruit last.

(It helps a lot to blend fruits with liquid first before adding other ingredients. Check beginning of each section for special instructions)

2. Blend on medium and increase to high for 1 minute. Repeat as necessary.

BEET HAPPY JUICE

Ingredients
3 whole beets, stems removed & cut in half
1 green apple – quartered & seeded
1/2 lemon
thumb size of ginger

Directions:
1. Add liquid first, then softer ingredients and harder items like ice or frozen fruit last.

(It helps a lot to blend fruits with liquid first before adding other ingredients. Check beginning of each section for special instructions)

2. Blend on medium and increase to high for 1 minute. Repeat as necessary.

WATERMELON JUICE

Ingredients
1 small sweet, organic watermelon (a 6 pounder will do)
1 small lime, juiced

Directions:
1. Add liquid first, then softer ingredients and harder items like ice or frozen fruit last.

(It helps a lot to blend fruits with liquid first before adding other ingredients. Check beginning of each section for special instructions)

2. Blend on medium and increase to high for 1 minute. Repeat as necessary.

WATERMELON RASPBERRY LIME JUICE

Ingredients
½ smallish watermelon, seedless

3 - 4 ounces raspberries
2 limes, freshly squeezed
Directions:
1. Add liquid first, then softer ingredients and harder items like ice or frozen fruit last.

(It helps a lot to blend fruits with liquid first before adding other ingredients. Check beginning of each section for special instructions)
2. Blend on medium and increase to high for 1 minute. Repeat as necessary.

FRESH STRAWBERRY JUICE WITH COCONUT WATER

Ingredients
3 cups fresh organic strawberries, stems removed
1 organic pear, cored and seeded
1/4 fresh lime
small piece of ginger
1/2 cup coconut water
Directions:
1. Add liquid first, then softer ingredients and harder items like ice or frozen fruit last.

(It helps a lot to blend fruits with liquid first before adding other ingredients. Check beginning of each section for special instructions)
2. Blend on medium and increase to high for 1 minute. Repeat as necessary.

PURPLE RAIN DETOX JUICE

Ingredients
2 Fuji Apples
1 Beet with stalk
3 Kale Leaves
1 Cucumber
Directions:
1. Add liquid first, then softer ingredients and harder items like ice or frozen fruit last.

(It helps a lot to blend fruits with liquid first before adding other ingredients.

Check beginning of each section for special instructions)
2. Blend on medium and increase to high for 1 minute. Repeat as necessary.

GINGER CUCUMBER DETOX JUICE

Ingredients
2 cucumbers
2 inch knob of ginger
1/2 lime
1 cup of parsley
dash of cayenne pepper
Directions:
1. Add liquid first, then softer ingredients and harder items like ice or frozen fruit last.

(It helps a lot to blend fruits with liquid first before adding other ingredients. Check beginning of each section for special instructions)
2. Blend on medium and increase to high for 1 minute. Repeat as necessary.

PINA COLADA PINEAPPLE DETOX JUICE

Ingredients
One third of a large pineapple (about 400g)
2 apples
2 peaches
A thumb sized piece of root ginger
Directions:
1. Add liquid first, then softer ingredients and harder items like ice or frozen fruit last.

(It helps a lot to blend fruits with liquid first before adding other ingredients. Check beginning of each section for special instructions)
2. Blend on medium and increase to high for 1 minute. Repeat as necessary.

HOLLY'S GREEN JUICE

Ingredients

1 cucumber, peeled
1 handful of baby kale, or 1 kale stalk with stalk removed
1 handful of baby spinach
1 crown of broccoli
3 gala apples, peeled
Directions:
 1. Add liquid first, then softer ingredients and harder items like ice or frozen fruit last.
 (It helps a lot to blend fruits with liquid first before adding other ingredients. Check beginning of each section for special instructions)
 2. Blend on medium and increase to high for 1 minute. Repeat as necessary.

PEAR AND CARROT DETOX JUICE

Ingredients
2 pears (cored)
2 carrots
2 stalks celery
2 nectarines (pits removed)
1 lemon (remove the rind leaving most of the white on)
2 cups honeydew melon cubed
1 orange (remove rind leaving most of the white on)
1 inch piece ginger
Directions:
 1. Add liquid first, then softer ingredients and harder items like ice or frozen fruit last.
 (It helps a lot to blend fruits with liquid first before adding other ingredients. Check beginning of each section for special instructions)
2.   Blend on medium and increase to high for 1 minute. Repeat as necessary.

GREEN JUICE

Ingredients
2 bunches of curly kale
4 Fuji Apples

2 Lemons, skin removed
2 large cucumbers
1.5-2 inch slice of ginger, skin removed
Directions:
 1. Add liquid first, then softer ingredients and harder items like ice or frozen fruit last.
 (It helps a lot to blend fruits with liquid first before adding other ingredients. Check beginning of each section for special instructions)
 2. Blend on medium and increase to high for 1 minute. Repeat as necessary.

GINGER BEET JUICE

Ingredients
2 Small Beets (1.5 lbs) & the Beet Greens
2 Large Apples (the sweeter the better)
1 Small Lime
2 Clementines
1 Piece Fresh Ginger (about the size of your thumb)
1-2 Carrots (optional)
Directions:
 1. Add liquid first, then softer ingredients and harder items like ice or frozen fruit last.
 (It helps a lot to blend fruits with liquid first before adding other ingredients. Check beginning of each section for special instructions)
 2. Blend on medium and increase to high for 1 minute. Repeat as necessary.

KALE GRAPE GINGER LEMON JUICE

Ingredients
1 bunch organic kale
1 cup organic grapes
1 slice ginger, optional
juice of one lemon wedge
Directions:

1. Add liquid first, then softer ingredients and harder items like ice or frozen fruit last.

(It helps a lot to blend fruits with liquid first before adding other ingredients. Check beginning of each section for special instructions)

2. Blend on medium and increase to high for 1 minute. Repeat as necessary.

PEACHY KEEN

Ingredients
4 Sprigs Fresh Basil
½ - 1 Lemon
4 Peaches
8-10 Carrots
Directions:
1. Add liquid first, then softer ingredients and harder items like ice or frozen fruit last.

(It helps a lot to blend fruits with liquid first before adding other ingredients. Check beginning of each section for special instructions)

2. Blend on medium and increase to high for 1 minute. Repeat as necessary.

FENNEL & APPLE DETOX GREEN JUICE

Ingredients
1 bunch of spinach, washed (10 ounces)
1 bunch of mint
1 cucumber
2 green apples, cored
1 fennel bulb
½ lemon
Directions:
1. Add liquid first, then softer ingredients and harder items like ice or frozen fruit last.

(It helps a lot to blend fruits with liquid first before adding other ingredients. Check beginning of each section for special instructions)

2. Blend on medium and increase to high for 1 minute. Repeat as necessary.

ORANGE CREAM JUICE

Ingredients
1 small cooked sweet potato
2 large carrots
3 clementines (peeled)
1/2 cup almond milk (original or vanilla)
Directions:
1. Add liquid first, then softer ingredients and harder items like ice or frozen fruit last.

(It helps a lot to blend fruits with liquid first before adding other ingredients. Check beginning of each section for special instructions)

2. Blend on medium and increase to high for 1 minute. Repeat as necessary.

RICKI HELLER'S CRANBERRY, POMEGRANATE HOLIDAY DETOX JUICE

Ingredients
4-6 large leaves kale
1 cup pomegranate arils (from one large ripe pomegranate)
1 cup fresh or frozen cranberries (if frozen, thaw before juicing)
1 pear, cored
1 knob (about 1 inch or 2.5 cm) fresh ginger, peeled
6-12 leaves of fresh mint, optional
stevia, to taste
Directions:
1. Add liquid first, then softer ingredients and harder items like ice or frozen fruit last.

(It helps a lot to blend fruits with liquid first before adding other ingredients. Check beginning of each section for special instructions)

2. Blend on medium and increase to high for 1 minute. Repeat as necessary.

CARROT GINGER JUICE

Ingredients

2 cups chopped and peeled carrots (about four large carrots)
2 cups cold water
4 tbsps chopped and peeled fresh ginger root (about one three inch piece)
1 tbsp fresh lemon juice (the juice of half of one small lemon)

Directions:

1. Add liquid first, then softer ingredients and harder items like ice or frozen fruit last.
(It helps a lot to blend fruits with liquid first before adding other ingredients. Check beginning of each section for special instructions)
2. Blend on medium and increase to high for 1 minute. Repeat as necessary.

BROCCOLI JUICE

Ingredients

4 carrots (smaller)
6 strawberries
1 broccoli stalk

Directions:

1. Add liquid first, then softer ingredients and harder items like ice or frozen fruit last.
(It helps a lot to blend fruits with liquid first before adding other ingredients. Check beginning of each section for special instructions)
2. Blend on medium and increase to high for 1 minute. Repeat as necessary.

CLASSIC BEET JUICE

Ingredients

1 red beet, peel on, chopped
1 fuji apple, cored and chopped (peel on)
1 kale leaf, stem removed and discarded
1 orange, peeled and squeezed
1 teaspoon orange rind
1 teaspoon grated ginger
1-1/2 cups coconut water

Directions:

1. Add liquid first, then softer ingredients and harder items like ice or frozen fruit last.
(It helps a lot to blend fruits with liquid first before adding other ingredients. Check beginning of each section for special instructions)
2. Blend on medium and increase to high for 1 minute. Repeat as necessary.

PLUM AND GINGER DETOX JUICE

Ingredients

6 to 8 cup of plums, deseeded and chopped
2 inch piece of ginger, chopped
1 teaspoon of kala namak or black salt
honey or sugar to taste

Directions:

1. Add liquid first, then softer ingredients and harder items like ice or frozen fruit last.
(It helps a lot to blend fruits with liquid first before adding other ingredients. Check beginning of each section for special instructions)
2. Blend on medium and increase to high for 1 minute. Repeat as necessary.

GREEN JUICE FOR BEGINNERS

Ingredients

4 black dino kale leaves
1/3 pineapple
2 red delicious apples
1 lime
1" knob of ginger
1 handful Italian parsley

Directions:

1. Add liquid first, then softer ingredients and harder items like ice or frozen fruit last.
(It helps a lot to blend fruits with liquid first before adding other ingredients.

Check beginning of each section for
special instructions)
 2. Blend on medium and increase to
high for 1 minute. Repeat as necessary.

LEAN & MEAN GREEN JUICE

Ingredients
5 romaine leaves
5 kale leaves
1 cucumber, peeled
1/2 bunch parsley
3 celery stalks
1 cup green grapes
Directions:
 1. Add liquid first, then softer
ingredients and harder items like ice or
frozen fruit last.
 (It helps a lot to blend fruits with liquid
first before adding other ingredients.
Check beginning of each section for
special instructions)
 2. Blend on medium and increase to
high for 1 minute. Repeat as necessary.

PRIMAVERA GREEN JUICE

Ingredients
2 green apples, halved and quartered
4 stalks celery
1 cucumber, peeled
6 romaine leaves
5 kale leaves
1 lemon, peeled
Directions:
 1. Add liquid first, then softer
ingredients and harder items like ice or
frozen fruit last.
 (It helps a lot to blend fruits with liquid
first before adding other ingredients.
Check beginning of each section for
special instructions)
 2. Blend on medium and increase to
high for 1 minute. Repeat as necessary.

POPEYE POTION

Ingredients
2 very large fistfuls of spinach

1/2 cucumber
2 apples
thumb size piece ginger
1/2 lemon
Directions:
 1. Add liquid first, then softer
ingredients and harder items like ice or
frozen fruit last.
 (It helps a lot to blend fruits with liquid
first before adding other ingredients.
Check beginning of each section for
special instructions)
 2. Blend on medium and increase to
high for 1 minute. Repeat as necessary.

PINEAPPLE GREEN JUICE

Ingredients
1 cup Pineapple
1 Granny Smith Apple
1 Large Broccoli Stalk and florets
5 Kale Leaves
1 cup Spinach
Large handful Fresh Mint
Directions:
 1. Add liquid first, then softer
ingredients and harder items like ice or
frozen fruit last.
 (It helps a lot to blend fruits with liquid
first before adding other ingredients.
Check beginning of each section for
special instructions)
 2. Blend on medium and increase to
high for 1 minute. Repeat as necessary.

GREEN GODDESS JUICE

Ingredients
2 cups pineapple, cut into chunks (1/2 a
small pineapple)
1 1/2 cups broccoli, cut into chunks
1 large cucumber, sliced
3 handfuls of spinach
1 handful of mint
1 lemon, juice reserved
Directions:

1. Add liquid first, then softer
ingredients and harder items like ice or
frozen fruit last.
 (It helps a lot to blend fruits with liquid
first before adding other ingredients.
Check beginning of each section for
special instructions)
 2. Blend on medium and increase to
high for 1 minute. Repeat as necessary.

BEET COCONUT JUICE AND JUICING WITHOUT A JUICER

Ingredients
1 red beet, peel on, chopped
1 fuji apple, cored and chopped (peel on)
1 la;e leaf, stem removed and discarded
1 orange, peeled and squeezed
1 teaspoon orange rind
1 teaspoon grated ginger
1-½ cups coconut water
Directions:
 1. Add liquid first, then softer
ingredients and harder items like ice or
frozen fruit last.
 (It helps a lot to blend fruits with liquid
first before adding other ingredients.
Check beginning of each section for
special instructions)
 2. Blend on medium and increase to
high for 1 minute. Repeat as necessary.

GREEN JUICE II

Ingredients
½ red grapefruit
about 4 chunks of pineapple
handful of spinach
handful of parsley
2 large stick of celery
Directions:
 1. Add liquid first, then softer
ingredients and harder items like ice or
frozen fruit last.
 (It helps a lot to blend fruits with liquid
first before adding other ingredients.

Check beginning of each section for
special instructions)
 2. Blend on medium and increase to
high for 1 minute. Repeat as necessary.

SWEET FREEDOM'S GREEN JUICE

Ingredients
2 carrots
2 green apples
2 kiwis
½ a cucumber
2-3 handfuls of spinach
a small bunch of kale or swiss chard, or
any green really
2-3 leaves of romaine lettuce
1 lemon
a nub of ginger, peeled
water to dilute (optional)
Directions:
 1. Add liquid first, then softer
ingredients and harder items like ice or
frozen fruit last.
 (It helps a lot to blend fruits with liquid
first before adding other ingredients.
Check beginning of each section for
special instructions)
 2. Blend on medium and increase to
high for 1 minute. Repeat as necessary.

FEEL BETTER GREEN JUICE

Ingredients
1 green apple, seeds removed
1 orange, peeled
1 stalk celery
½" piece of fresh ginger
1 large carrot
Freshly squeezed lemon juice to taste
Directions:
 1. Add liquid first, then softer
ingredients and harder items like ice or
frozen fruit last.
 (It helps a lot to blend fruits with liquid
first before adding other ingredients.

Check beginning of each section for special instructions)
 2. Blend on medium and increase to high for 1 minute. Repeat as necessary.

STAY HEALTHY GREEN JUICE

Ingredients
3 leaves kale
1 apple, core removed
½ inch fresh ginger
1 cup spinach
1 small cucumber
Juice of ½ lemon
4 sprigs cilantro
1 cup water
Directions:
 1. Add liquid first, then softer ingredients and harder items like ice or frozen fruit last.
 (It helps a lot to blend fruits with liquid first before adding other ingredients. Check beginning of each section for special instructions)
 2. Blend on medium and increase to high for 1 minute. Repeat as necessary.

HIPPIE JUICE

Ingredients
1 cup Watermelon juice
⅓ cup kale
⅓ cup coconut water
4 scoops Pink Lemonade mix
Water
Strawberries
Directions:
 1. Add liquid first, then softer ingredients and harder items like ice or frozen fruit last.
 (It helps a lot to blend fruits with liquid first before adding other ingredients. Check beginning of each section for special instructions)
 2. Blend on medium and increase to high for 1 minute. Repeat as necessary.

GRAPEFRUIT STRAWBERRY JUICE

Ingredients
3 grapefruits, lightly peeled
2 cups strawberries, roughly chopped
2 tbsp Stevia powder,
or sweetener of choice
Directions:
 1. Add liquid first, then softer ingredients and harder items like ice or frozen fruit last.
 (It helps a lot to blend fruits with liquid first before adding other ingredients. Check beginning of each section for special instructions)
 2. Blend on medium and increase to high for 1 minute. Repeat as necessary.

CARROT APPLE GLOW JUICE

Ingredients
2 large organic carrots, tops trimmed
1 organic Granny Smith apple, cut into quarters
1 Navel orange, quartered and peeled
Directions:
 1. Add liquid first, then softer ingredients and harder items like ice or frozen fruit last.
 (It helps a lot to blend fruits with liquid first before adding other ingredients. Check beginning of each section for special instructions)
 2. Blend on medium and increase to high for 1 minute. Repeat as necessary.

BEET & BERRY LIVER CLEANSE JUICE

Ingredients
2 medium beets
2 c. blueberries
1 apple
2 large carrots
1/2 c. raw broccoli
1 whole lemon

2" knob ginger, skin removed
1/2-1 c. pure coconut water
Directions:
 1. Add liquid first, then softer ingredients and harder items like ice or frozen fruit last.
 (It helps a lot to blend fruits with liquid first before adding other ingredients. Check beginning of each section for special instructions)
 2. Blend on medium and increase to high for 1 minute. Repeat as necessary.

BEET CARROT LEMON APPLE KALE CELERY GINGER JUICE

Ingredients
2 beets
3 carrots
1 lemon
1 apple
5 kale leaves
4 stalks celery
1 inch ginger
Directions:
 1. Add liquid first, then softer ingredients and harder items like ice or frozen fruit last.
 (It helps a lot to blend fruits with liquid first before adding other ingredients. Check beginning of each section for special instructions)
 2. Blend on medium and increase to high for 1 minute. Repeat as necessary.

PINEAPPLE GINGER PARADISE

Ingredients
½ a pineapple, skin cut off with a kitchen knife
½ a ripe mango, peeled
1 apple
½ a lime (skin on)
1” piece of peeled fresh ginger
Directions:

 1. Add liquid first, then softer ingredients and harder items like ice or frozen fruit last.
 (It helps a lot to blend fruits with liquid first before adding other ingredients. Check beginning of each section for special instructions)
 2. Blend on medium and increase to high for 1 minute. Repeat as necessary.

BEETROOT JUICE

Ingredients
1 small beetroot
1 stalk of celery
2 carrots
1 apple
2 leaves of Kale
Directions:
 1. Add liquid first, then softer ingredients and harder items like ice or frozen fruit last.
 (It helps a lot to blend fruits with liquid first before adding other ingredients. Check beginning of each section for special instructions)
 2. Blend on medium and increase to high for 1 minute. Repeat as necessary.

BUSY BEE DETOX JUICE

Ingredients
2 medium carrots
1 lemon - peeled
1” piece of ginger
1 stalk of celery
½ an apple
2 tbsp unfiltered apple cider vinegar
1 tsp organic bee pollen*
Directions:
 1. Add liquid first, then softer ingredients and harder items like ice or frozen fruit last.
 (It helps a lot to blend fruits with liquid first before adding other ingredients. Check beginning of each section for special instructions)

2. Blend on medium and increase to high for 1 minute. Repeat as necessary.

MIDNIGHT JUICE

Ingredients
1 cup Pomegranate Seeds
1 cup Cranberries
2 Valencia Oranges, peeled
1 Lime
Directions:
1. Add liquid first, then softer ingredients and harder items like ice or frozen fruit last.
(It helps a lot to blend fruits with liquid first before adding other ingredients. Check beginning of each section for special instructions)
2. Blend on medium and increase to high for 1 minute. Repeat as necessary.

EVERYDAY DETOX JUICE

Ingredients
1 quarter fresh pineapple
1 orange
½ handful cilantro
½ small jalapeño, seeded
Directions:
1. Add liquid first, then softer ingredients and harder items like ice or frozen fruit last.
(It helps a lot to blend fruits with liquid first before adding other ingredients. Check beginning of each section for special instructions)
2. Blend on medium and increase to high for 1 minute. Repeat as necessary.

GREEN DETOX JUICE

Ingredients
3 large kale leaves, washed
½ inch chunk of fresh ginger, peeled
2 celery stalks, washed
½ cup fresh parsley
1 small lemon (or ½ large lemon), peeled
1 cucumber, washed

2 small pears (or one large), washed and cored
Directions:
1. Add liquid first, then softer ingredients and harder items like ice or frozen fruit last.
(It helps a lot to blend fruits with liquid first before adding other ingredients. Check beginning of each section for special instructions)
2. Blend on medium and increase to high for 1 minute. Repeat as necessary.

LIVER DETOX JUICE

Ingredients
2 small beets
1 fennel bulb
2 carrots
1 lime
Directions:
1. Add liquid first, then softer ingredients and harder items like ice or frozen fruit last.
(It helps a lot to blend fruits with liquid first before adding other ingredients. Check beginning of each section for special instructions)
2. Blend on medium and increase to high for 1 minute. Repeat as necessary.

BLOOD ORANGE CHILI JUICE

Ingredients
6 Blood Oranges
2 Serrano Chili
Agave Nectar
Directions:
1. Add liquid first, then softer ingredients and harder items like ice or frozen fruit last.
(It helps a lot to blend fruits with liquid first before adding other ingredients. Check beginning of each section for special instructions)
2. Blend on medium and increase to high for 1 minute. Repeat as necessary.

PINEAPPLE DETOX JUICE

Ingredients
2-3 thick slices of fresh pineapple (the canned kind has tons of added sugars)
½ cucumber
⅓ cup aloe vera juice
½ cup coconut water
Directions:
 1. Add liquid first, then softer ingredients and harder items like ice or frozen fruit last.
 (It helps a lot to blend fruits with liquid first before adding other ingredients. Check beginning of each section for special instructions)
 2. Blend on medium and increase to high for 1 minute. Repeat as necessary.

SPINACH SHOTS

Ingredients
3 large handfuls spinach
⅓ of a lemon, with peel (if it's organic)
1 green apple
Directions:
 1. Add liquid first, then softer ingredients and harder items like ice or frozen fruit last.
 (It helps a lot to blend fruits with liquid first before adding other ingredients. Check beginning of each section for special instructions)
 2. Blend on medium and increase to high for 1 minute. Repeat as necessary.

RED REVIVER

Ingredients
1 carrot
1 small beet
1 small ripe tomato
1 - 2 ½ inch wedge red cabbage
½ red bell pepper
¾ cup diced fresh pineapple
1 packet Monk Fruit In The Raw
½ cup cold water (optional)
Directions:

 1. Add liquid first, then softer ingredients and harder items like ice or frozen fruit last.
 (It helps a lot to blend fruits with liquid first before adding other ingredients. Check beginning of each section for special instructions)
 2. Blend on medium and increase to high for 1 minute. Repeat as necessary.

ORANGE BROCCOLI JUICE

Ingredients
2 apples
1 stalk broccoli
4 carrots
Directions:
 1. Add liquid first, then softer ingredients and harder items like ice or frozen fruit last.
 (It helps a lot to blend fruits with liquid first before adding other ingredients. Check beginning of each section for special instructions)
 2. Blend on medium and increase to high for 1 minute. Repeat as necessary.

GREEN GUNSLINGER

Ingredients
2 peeled kiwi
2 green apples
1 cucumber
1 cup fresh spinach
Directions:
 1. Add liquid first, then softer ingredients and harder items like ice or frozen fruit last.
 (It helps a lot to blend fruits with liquid first before adding other ingredients. Check beginning of each section for special instructions)
 2. Blend on medium and increase to high for 1 minute. Repeat as necessary.

RHUBARB JUICE

Ingredients
2 pounds rhubarb stalks

8 cups water
Directions:
 1. Add liquid first, then softer ingredients and harder items like ice or frozen fruit last.
 (It helps a lot to blend fruits with liquid first before adding other ingredients. Check beginning of each section for special instructions)
 2. Blend on medium and increase to high for 1 minute. Repeat as necessary.

CRANBERRY POMEGRANATE AND KALE JUICE

Ingredients
4-6 large leaves kale
1 cup pomegranate arils (from one large ripe pomegranate)
1 cup fresh or frozen cranberries (if frozen, thaw before juicing)
1 pear, cored
1 knob (about 1 inch or 2.5 cm) fresh ginger, peeled
6-12 leaves of fresh mint, optional
stevia, to taste
Directions:
 1. Add liquid first, then softer ingredients and harder items like ice or frozen fruit last.
 (It helps a lot to blend fruits with liquid first before adding other ingredients. Check beginning of each section for special instructions)
 2. Blend on medium and increase to high for 1 minute. Repeat as necessary.

SPICED APPLE CIDER JUICE

Ingredients
3 large apples, cored and chopped
1/2 teaspoon of ground cinnamon
1/4 teaspoon of ground nutmeg
Directions:
 1. Add liquid first, then softer ingredients and harder items like ice or frozen fruit last.

 (It helps a lot to blend fruits with liquid first before adding other ingredients. Check beginning of each section for special instructions)
 2. Blend on medium and increase to high for 1 minute. Repeat as necessary.

TOMATO WITH A KICK

Ingredients
2 tomatoes
2 green lettuce leaves
2 radishes
4 parsley sprigs
½ lemon
Directions:
 1. Add liquid first, then softer ingredients and harder items like ice or frozen fruit last.
 (It helps a lot to blend fruits with liquid first before adding other ingredients. Check beginning of each section for special instructions)
 2. Blend on medium and increase to high for 1 minute. Repeat as necessary.

ENERGIZER BUNNY ON CRACK JUICE

Ingredients
3 kale leaves and stalk
1/2 cucumber
1/2 cup spinach
3 stalks of celery
1/4 fennel bulb
1/4 head of romaine lettuce (or napa cabbage)
1-2 apples
1/2 inch ginger
Directions:
 1. Add liquid first, then softer ingredients and harder items like ice or frozen fruit last.
 (It helps a lot to blend fruits with liquid first before adding other ingredients. Check beginning of each section for special instructions)

2. Blend on medium and increase to high for 1 minute. Repeat as necessary.

SWEET CURB APPETITE JUICE

Ingredients
1 large sweet potato
2-3 carrots
1 orange
¼ pineapple (about 1 cup chopped pineapples)
optional: squeeze half a lemon in
Directions:
1. Add liquid first, then softer ingredients and harder items like ice or frozen fruit last.
(It helps a lot to blend fruits with liquid first before adding other ingredients. Check beginning of each section for special instructions)
2. Blend on medium and increase to high for 1 minute. Repeat as necessary.

GREEN GUT BEGONE!

Ingredients
5 celery stalks
2 kale stalks
6-8 romaine leaves (or napa cabbage)
1 apple
palmful of parsley
½ knob of ginger
Directions:
1. Add liquid first, then softer ingredients and harder items like ice or frozen fruit last.
(It helps a lot to blend fruits with liquid first before adding other ingredients. Check beginning of each section for special instructions)
2. Blend on medium and increase to high for 1 minute. Repeat as necessary.

BEET BLOOD INFUSION JUICE

Ingredients
½ small beet

3 chard leaves (or kale)
2 cucumbers
1 apple
pinch of cayenne pepper
Directions:
1. Add liquid first, then softer ingredients and harder items like ice or frozen fruit last.
(It helps a lot to blend fruits with liquid first before adding other ingredients. Check beginning of each section for special instructions)
2. Blend on medium and increase to high for 1 minute. Repeat as necessary.

STRONG CORE JUICE

Ingredients
2 cups spinach
1 broccoli floret
1 cucumber
handful of parsley
1 lemon
1/2 inch ginger
Directions:
1. Add liquid first, then softer ingredients and harder items like ice or frozen fruit last.
(It helps a lot to blend fruits with liquid first before adding other ingredients. Check beginning of each section for special instructions)
2. Blend on medium and increase to high for 1 minute. Repeat as necessary.

MEAN GREEN JUICE

Ingredients
1 cucumber
4 celery stalks
2 apples
6-8 leaves kale
1/2 lemon
1 in (2.5 cm) piece of ginger
Directions:

1. Add liquid first, then softer ingredients and harder items like ice or frozen fruit last.

(It helps a lot to blend fruits with liquid first before adding other ingredients. Check beginning of each section for special instructions)

2. Blend on medium and increase to high for 1 minute. Repeat as necessary.

BRIGHT-EYED GREEN JUICE

Ingredients

5 small carrots
1 large cucumber
3 handfuls cilantro
2 handfuls kale
1 small lime

Directions:

1. Add liquid first, then softer ingredients and harder items like ice or frozen fruit last.

(It helps a lot to blend fruits with liquid first before adding other ingredients. Check beginning of each section for special instructions)

2. Blend on medium and increase to high for 1 minute. Repeat as necessary.

IRON AND VITAMIN C BOOSTING GREEN JUICE

Ingredients

½ field cucumber
1 cup green grapes
½ cup spinach
2 small kiwis
1-2 cups of water

Directions:

1. Add liquid first, then softer ingredients and harder items like ice or frozen fruit last.

(It helps a lot to blend fruits with liquid first before adding other ingredients. Check beginning of each section for special instructions)

2. Blend on medium and increase to high for 1 minute. Repeat as necessary.

FAT DISSOLVER JUICE

Ingredients

1 pink grapefruit, peeled
2 oranges, peeled
1 bunch mint
1 head romaine lettuce

Directions:

1. Add liquid first, then softer ingredients and harder items like ice or frozen fruit last.

(It helps a lot to blend fruits with liquid first before adding other ingredients. Check beginning of each section for special instructions)

2. Blend on medium and increase to high for 1 minute. Repeat as necessary.

SKIN REJUVENATING GREEN JUICE

Ingredients

1 cup blackberries
4 sprigs mint
½ fennel bulb with greens
2 stalks kale
2 small green apples
1 cup broccoli
1 handful watercress
1 small cucumber
1 lemon, peeled

Directions:

1. Add liquid first, then softer ingredients and harder items like ice or frozen fruit last.

(It helps a lot to blend fruits with liquid first before adding other ingredients. Check beginning of each section for special instructions)

2. Blend on medium and increase to high for 1 minute. Repeat as necessary.

LEAN GREEN POWER JUICE

Ingredients

½ pineapple, peeled, cored and chopped
½ english cucumber, peeled and chopped
½ ripe pear, peeled, cored and chopped
juice from 1 lime
1 cup baby spinach leaves
10 mint leaves, chopped
1 tsp agave nectar
crushed ice
Directions:
 1. Add liquid first, then softer ingredients and harder items like ice or frozen fruit last.
 (It helps a lot to blend fruits with liquid first before adding other ingredients. Check beginning of each section for special instructions)
 2. Blend on medium and increase to high for 1 minute. Repeat as necessary.

HEALTHY COLADA GREEN JUICE RECIPE

Ingredients
1 cucumber
1 heart of romaine lettuce
3 celery sticks
4 cups ripe pineapple
1-inch piece ginger
1/2 cup coconut water
Directions:
 1. Add liquid first, then softer ingredients and harder items like ice or frozen fruit last.
 (It helps a lot to blend fruits with liquid first before adding other ingredients. Check beginning of each section for special instructions)
 2. Blend on medium and increase to high for 1 minute. Repeat as necessary.

THINK GREEN JUICE

Ingredients
1 celery stalk with leaves, chopped
1 green apple, cored and chopped

2 large kale leaves, stems removed
1 cucumber, chopped
1/2 inch piece of ginger, chopped
handful of spinach leaves
handful of mint leaves
juice of 2 limes
2 teaspoons stevia (or raw sugar)
1/4 teaspoon salt flakes
600ml cold water
1 teaspoon spirulina powder (optional)
Directions:
 1. Add liquid first, then softer ingredients and harder items like ice or frozen fruit last.
 (It helps a lot to blend fruits with liquid first before adding other ingredients. Check beginning of each section for special instructions)
 2. Blend on medium and increase to high for 1 minute. Repeat as necessary.

BLUEPEARY JUICE

Ingredients
2 ripe pears
2 cups spinach or baby spinach
1 cups blueberries
Directions:
 1. Add liquid first, then softer ingredients and harder items like ice or frozen fruit last.
 (It helps a lot to blend fruits with liquid first before adding other ingredients. Check beginning of each section for special instructions)
 2. Blend on medium and increase to high for 1 minute. Repeat as necessary.

MAGENTA ZING

Ingredients
Watermelon (1/4 of a small size watermelon)
Apples - 2
Carrots - 4
Beets - 1 with leaves
Celery - 3 stalks

Ginger - 1 inch
Directions:
 1. Add liquid first, then softer
ingredients and harder items like ice or
frozen fruit last.
 (It helps a lot to blend fruits with liquid
first before adding other ingredients.
Check beginning of each section for
special instructions)
 2. Blend on medium and increase to
high for 1 minute. Repeat as necessary.

DARK KNIGHT

Ingredients
Apples - 2
Cucumber - 1
Baby Celery - 1/2 bunch
Carrots - 3
Spinach - about 1/2 bunch
Swiss Chard - 3 stalks
Directions:
 1. Add liquid first, then softer
ingredients and harder items like ice or
frozen fruit last.
 (It helps a lot to blend fruits with liquid
first before adding other ingredients.
Check beginning of each section for
special instructions)
 2. Blend on medium and increase to
high for 1 minute. Repeat as necessary.

LEFTOVERS

Ingredients
Strawberries - about 15
Pineapples - 3 spears
Watermelon - very little
Celery - 3 stalks
Cucumber - 1/4
Carrots - 2
Dino Kale - 3 leaves
Spinach - about 1/2 bunch
Directions:
 1. Add liquid first, then softer
ingredients and harder items like ice or
frozen fruit last.

 (It helps a lot to blend fruits with liquid
first before adding other ingredients.
Check beginning of each section for
special instructions)
 2. Blend on medium and increase to
high for 1 minute. Repeat as necessary.

CITRUS SENSATION

Ingredients
Pineapple - 2 spears
Oranges - 2 to 3
Strawberries - handful
Lemon - 1
Apples – 2
Directions:
 1. Add liquid first, then softer
ingredients and harder items like ice or
frozen fruit last.
 (It helps a lot to blend fruits with liquid
first before adding other ingredients.
Check beginning of each section for
special instructions)
 2. Blend on medium and increase to
high for 1 minute. Repeat as necessary.

BRIGHT GREEN GOODNESS

Ingredients
Spinach - 1/2 bunch
Dino kale - 8 leaves
Cucumber - 1/2
Celery - 4 to 5
Baby celery
Pineapple core
Ginger - 1/2 inch
Directions:
 1. Add liquid first, then softer
ingredients and harder items like ice or
frozen fruit last.
 (It helps a lot to blend fruits with liquid
first before adding other ingredients.
Check beginning of each section for
special instructions)
 2. Blend on medium and increase to
high for 1 minute. Repeat as necessary.

DELICIOUS MINT REFRESHER

Ingredients
Pineapples spears - 4
Strawberries - 1 handful
Apple - 1
Mint leaves - about 30
Directions:
1. Add liquid first, then softer ingredients and harder items like ice or frozen fruit last.
(It helps a lot to blend fruits with liquid first before adding other ingredients. Check beginning of each section for special instructions)
2. Blend on medium and increase to high for 1 minute. Repeat as necessary.

MANGO TANGO

Ingredients
Pineapple - 2 spears
Strawberries - 7
Mango - 1
Nectarine - 1
Apple - 1
Orange – 1
Directions:
1. Add liquid first, then softer ingredients and harder items like ice or frozen fruit last.
(It helps a lot to blend fruits with liquid first before adding other ingredients. Check beginning of each section for special instructions)
2. Blend on medium and increase to high for 1 minute. Repeat as necessary.

GREEN AND ORANGE POWER

Ingredients
Spinach - 1/2 bunch
Carrots - 6
Golden beets - 1
Apple - 1
Lemon - 1
Orange – 1

Directions:
1. Add liquid first, then softer ingredients and harder items like ice or frozen fruit last.
(It helps a lot to blend fruits with liquid first before adding other ingredients. Check beginning of each section for special instructions)
2. Blend on medium and increase to high for 1 minute. Repeat as necessary.

RED CARROT ENVY

Ingredients
Red carrots - 3
Oranges - 1
Apple - 1
Cucumber - 1/2
Baby celery
Directions:
1. Add liquid first, then softer ingredients and harder items like ice or frozen fruit last.
(It helps a lot to blend fruits with liquid first before adding other ingredients. Check beginning of each section for special instructions)
2. Blend on medium and increase to high for 1 minute. Repeat as necessary.

KALE SURPRISE

Ingredients
Nectarine - 1
Oranges - 2
Dino kale - 8 leaves
Red carrots - 2
Apple 1
Directions:
1. Add liquid first, then softer ingredients and harder items like ice or frozen fruit last.
(It helps a lot to blend fruits with liquid first before adding other ingredients. Check beginning of each section for special instructions)

2. Blend on medium and increase to high for 1 minute. Repeat as necessary.

MIRACLE CURE JUICE

Ingredients
2 large beets
4 long carrots
2 apples (of any kind)
6 stalks celery
2 limes
2 inches ginger
Directions:
1. Add liquid first, then softer ingredients and harder items like ice or frozen fruit last.
(It helps a lot to blend fruits with liquid first before adding other ingredients. Check beginning of each section for special instructions)
2. Blend on medium and increase to high for 1 minute. Repeat as necessary.

LIGHT AND LEMONY ALOE JUICE

Ingredients
1 Cucumber
1 Apple
1 Lemon
2 tbsp Aloe vera pulp
Directions:
1. Add liquid first, then softer ingredients and harder items like ice or frozen fruit last.
(It helps a lot to blend fruits with liquid first before adding other ingredients. Check beginning of each section for special instructions)
2. Blend on medium and increase to high for 1 minute. Repeat as necessary.

HEALTH ALOE JUICE

Ingredients
1 Cucumber
1 Apple
1 Lemon

2 tbsp Aloe vera pulp
Directions:
1. Add liquid first, then softer ingredients and harder items like ice or frozen fruit last.
(It helps a lot to blend fruits with liquid first before adding other ingredients. Check beginning of each section for special instructions)
2. Blend on medium and increase to high for 1 minute. Repeat as necessary.

EXOTIC ALOE VERA JUICE

Ingredients
1-2 cup Fresh pineapple
1 Carrot
1 Green apple
1 tbsp Aloe vera pulp
A few tbsp of coconut milk is optional
Directions:
1. Add liquid first, then softer ingredients and harder items like ice or frozen fruit last.
(It helps a lot to blend fruits with liquid first before adding other ingredients. Check beginning of each section for special instructions)
2. Blend on medium and increase to high for 1 minute. Repeat as necessary.

FRESH & FRUITY JUNGLE JUICE

Ingredients
6 cups of ice cubes
1 96 oz container of Tropical Punch Kool-Aid
1/2 container Orange Kool-Aid Liquid
1 bag of your favorite frozen fruit mix
Directions:
1. Add liquid first, then softer ingredients and harder items like ice or frozen fruit last.
(It helps a lot to blend fruits with liquid first before adding other ingredients.

Check beginning of each section for special instructions)

2. Blend on medium and increase to high for 1 minute. Repeat as necessary.

NO MORE SINUS

Ingredients

2 carrots
2 oranges
1 green apple
a small piece of ginger (optional)

Directions:

1. Add liquid first, then softer ingredients and harder items like ice or frozen fruit last.

(It helps a lot to blend fruits with liquid first before adding other ingredients. Check beginning of each section for special instructions)

2. Blend on medium and increase to high for 1 minute. Repeat as necessary.

CANCER FIGHTING GREEN JUICE

Ingredients

1 cup broccoli
1 cup cucumber
2 cup romaine lettuce
1/2 cup cilantro
1/2 green apple *optional
1 lime

Directions:

1. Add liquid first, then softer ingredients and harder items like ice or frozen fruit last.

(It helps a lot to blend fruits with liquid first before adding other ingredients. Check beginning of each section for special instructions)

2. Blend on medium and increase to high for 1 minute. Repeat as necessary.

ORANGE, SPINACH AND MINT

Ingredients

½ bunch of spinach

2 large navel oranges
2 mint leaves

Directions:

1. Add liquid first, then softer ingredients and harder items like ice or frozen fruit last.

(It helps a lot to blend fruits with liquid first before adding other ingredients. Check beginning of each section for special instructions)

2. Blend on medium and increase to high for 1 minute. Repeat as necessary.

LIVER CLEANSE GRAPE JUICE

Ingredients

Water - 4-8 ounces (boiled and cooled)
Fresh lemon – 1
Ginger root - 1 inch, thinly sliced
Grape juice
8 oz or 1 cup
Flaxseed oil (or extra virgin olive oil)- 1 tbsp (slightly increase the quantity every day)
Garlic cloves - 1 (increase by 1 clove each day)
Cumin powder - 3 to 4 pinches
Fresh Mint - 3 to 4 leaves (optional)

Directions:

1. Add liquid first, then softer ingredients and harder items like ice or frozen fruit last.

(It helps a lot to blend fruits with liquid first before adding other ingredients. Check beginning of each section for special instructions)

2. Blend on medium and increase to high for 1 minute. Repeat as necessary.

LIVER DETOXIFICATION VEGETABLE JUICE

Ingredients

Fresh cabbage - 125 g
Fresh lemon - 1
Celery - 25 g
Fresh pear - 250 g

Ginger root - 1 inch
Filtered Water - 500 ml
Fresh Mint - 4 to 5 leaves
Directions:
 1. Add liquid first, then softer
ingredients and harder items like ice or
frozen fruit last.
 (It helps a lot to blend fruits with liquid
first before adding other ingredients.
Check beginning of each section for
special instructions)
 2. Blend on medium and increase to
high for 1 minute. Repeat as necessary.

BELLY BUSTER GREEN JUICE

Ingredients
3 medium apples
1 large cucumber
1 large lemon, including skin
1 lime, including skin
3 small mandarins, including skin
1 head romaine lettuce
Directions:
 1. Add liquid first, then softer
ingredients and harder items like ice or
frozen fruit last.
 (It helps a lot to blend fruits with liquid
first before adding other ingredients.
Check beginning of each section for
special instructions)
 2. Blend on medium and increase to
high for 1 minute. Repeat as necessary.

REBOOT ESSENTIALS

Ingredients
1 apple (large or medium)
1 lemon
4 celery stalks
2 medium-large carrots
6-10 stems parsley
6-8 stems fresh mint
Directions:
 1. Add liquid first, then softer
ingredients and harder items like ice or
frozen fruit last.

 (It helps a lot to blend fruits with liquid
first before adding other ingredients.
Check beginning of each section for
special instructions)
 2. Blend on medium and increase to
high for 1 minute. Repeat as necessary.

25 Nut milk recipes

Directions:
1.   Soak the nuts in filtered water for 6-8 hours and rinse thoroughly.
2.   Blend the ingredients for the recipe you are making on high for 1 min.
3.   If you prefer nut milk without tiny nut bits, use a straining cloth to push the milk through
4.   Re-blend for 45 seconds to 1 min (also optional).
Tip: For best results, blend the nuts in liquid 1-2 cups at a time. This will help your blender completely blend all nut pieces.

PLAIN ALMOND MILK

Ingredients
1 cup soaked almonds
3-4 cups filtered water
Additional filtered water for soaking almonds
A sweetener such as 1-2 tbsp honey, maple syrup, agave, dates
(5 or so) stevia etc.
Optional flavorants such as cinnamon, vanilla, or cocoa
Directions:
 1. Add liquid first, then softer ingredients and harder items like ice or frozen fruit last.
 (It helps a lot to blend fruits with liquid first before adding other ingredients. Check beginning of each section for special instructions)
 2. Blend on medium and increase to high for 1 minute. Repeat as necessary.

EASY HOMEMADE HORCHATA

Ingredients
1 cup soaked cashews
2/3 cup white rice, uncooked (medium or long-grain preferred)
2 1/2 cups water (first blend)
3 cups water (second blend)
one 3-inch cinnamon stick
2/3 cup granulated sugar, or to taste*
1/2 teaspoon vanilla extract
Directions:
 1. Add liquid first, then softer ingredients and harder items like ice or frozen fruit last.
 (It helps a lot to blend fruits with liquid first before adding other ingredients. Check beginning of each section for special instructions)
 2. Blend on medium and increase to high for 1 minute. Repeat as necessary.

CASHEW MILK

Ingredients
1 cup soaked cashews
4 cups water (divided)
1 to 2 tbsps maple syrup or honey or agave nectar
2 teaspoons vanilla extract
dash sea salt
pinch cinnamon (optional)
Directions:
 1. Add liquid first, then softer ingredients and harder items like ice or frozen fruit last.
 (It helps a lot to blend fruits with liquid first before adding other ingredients. Check beginning of each section for special instructions)
 2. Blend on medium and increase to high for 1 minute. Repeat as necessary.

CASHEW MILK LATTES

Ingredients
1 1/2 cups hot cashew milk
1 cup brewed coffee (preferably strong coffee)
2-3 large Medjool dates, pitted and roughly chopped
1 teaspoon vanilla extract
pinch of ground cinnamon (to top with)

Directions:
 1. Add liquid first, then softer ingredients and harder items like ice or frozen fruit last.
 (It helps a lot to blend fruits with liquid first before adding other ingredients. Check beginning of each section for special instructions)
 2. Blend on medium and increase to high for 1 minute. Repeat as necessary.

RAW CACAO HAZELNUT MILK

Ingredients
1 cup soaked unsalted organic hazelnuts
4 cups filtered or purified water
pinch of himalayan sea salt
2 tbsps local raw honey or other sweetener
1 vanilla bean
2 tbsps raw cacao powder
Directions:
 1. Add liquid first, then softer ingredients and harder items like ice or frozen fruit last.
 (It helps a lot to blend fruits with liquid first before adding other ingredients. Check beginning of each section for special instructions)
 2. Blend on medium and increase to high for 1 minute. Repeat as necessary.

VANILLA CINNAMON ALMOND MILK

Ingredients
1 cup soaked almonds, soaked in water
3.5 cups filtered water
2-4 pitted Medjool dates*, to taste
1 whole vanilla bean, chopped (or 1/2-1 tsp vanilla extract)
1/4 teaspoon cinnamon
small pinch of fine grain sea salt, to enhance the flavor
Directions:

 1. Add liquid first, then softer ingredients and harder items like ice or frozen fruit last.
 (It helps a lot to blend fruits with liquid first before adding other ingredients. Check beginning of each section for special instructions)
 2. Blend on medium and increase to high for 1 minute. Repeat as necessary.

TURMERIC ALMOND MILK

Ingredients
1 cup organic soaked unsalted almonds
4 cups filtered or purified water
pinch of himalayan sea salt (optional)
1 tbsp local raw honey or other sweetener (optional)
1-2 tbsps turmeric powder (I find turmeric to have a mild flavor, so I go with 2 tbsps)
Directions:
 1. Add liquid first, then softer ingredients and harder items like ice or frozen fruit last.
 (It helps a lot to blend fruits with liquid first before adding other ingredients. Check beginning of each section for special instructions)
 2. Blend on medium and increase to high for 1 minute. Repeat as necessary.

NUT MILK WITH CHOCOLATE HAZELNUT AND HONEY CINNAMON CASHEW

Ingredients
1 cup soaked almonds, cashews, or hazelnuts
1 tbsp chia seeds
2 cups cold filtered water
2 cups coconut water
1-2 tbsps raw honey or 4 pitted dates soaked in warm water for about 5 minutes
1 teaspoon vanilla extract or 1/2 vanilla bean scraped

1 pinch fine sea salt
Directions:
 1. Add liquid first, then softer ingredients and harder items like ice or frozen fruit last.
 (It helps a lot to blend fruits with liquid first before adding other ingredients. Check beginning of each section for special instructions)
 2. Blend on medium and increase to high for 1 minute. Repeat as necessary.

HOMEMADE RAW VEGAN BRAZIL NUT MILK

Ingredients
1 cup soaked brazil nuts
4 cups filtered water
4 pitted dates
1 pinch sea salt
1 tsp vanilla extract
Directions:
 1. Add liquid first, then softer ingredients and harder items like ice or frozen fruit last.
 (It helps a lot to blend fruits with liquid first before adding other ingredients. Check beginning of each section for special instructions)
 2. Blend on medium and increase to high for 1 minute. Repeat as necessary.

PISTACHIO MILK

Ingredients
1 cup soaked unsalted organic pistachios
4 cups filtered or purified water
pinch of himalayan sea salt
1 tbsp local raw honey or other sweetener
1 vanilla bean or 1 teaspoon vanilla extract (optional)
Directions:
 1. Add liquid first, then softer ingredients and harder items like ice or frozen fruit last.

 (It helps a lot to blend fruits with liquid first before adding other ingredients. Check beginning of each section for special instructions)
 2. Blend on medium and increase to high for 1 minute. Repeat as necessary.

HOMEMADE PECAN MILK

Ingredients
1 cup soaked pecans
1 tsp vanilla extract
2 pitted dates OR 2 tbsp honey, agave, or maple syrup OR a dropper of liquid stevia (optional) tiny pinch of sea salt (the salt actually brings out the sweetness!)
5 cups water
Directions:
 1. Add liquid first, then softer ingredients and harder items like ice or frozen fruit last.
 (It helps a lot to blend fruits with liquid first before adding other ingredients. Check beginning of each section for special instructions)
 2. Blend on medium and increase to high for 1 minute. Repeat as necessary.

CASHEW CREAM

Ingredients
1 cup soaked cashews or macadamia nuts (120g)
1/3 cup to 3/4 cup water
Directions:
 1. Add liquid first, then softer ingredients and harder items like ice or frozen fruit last.
 (It helps a lot to blend fruits with liquid first before adding other ingredients. Check beginning of each section for special instructions)
 2. Blend on medium and increase to high for 1 minute. Repeat as necessary.

STRAWBERRY MACADAMIA NUT MILK

Ingredients

1 cup soaked macadamia nuts (or almonds, or brazil nuts)
4 cups filtered water
2-3 cups sliced fresh strawberries
4-6 Pitted medjool dates
1 tbsp raw honey or maple syrup
1 teaspoon vanilla extract
Pinch of sea salt

Directions:

1. Add liquid first, then softer ingredients and harder items like ice or frozen fruit last.

(It helps a lot to blend fruits with liquid first before adding other ingredients. Check beginning of each section for special instructions)

2. Blend on medium and increase to high for 1 minute. Repeat as necessary.

GREEN CASHEW NUT MILK

Ingredients

1 cup of soaked cashews
4 cups of filtered water
10-12 dates
1 vanilla bean
1/4 tsp sea salt
4 cups of spinach
4 cups of kale

Directions:

1. Add liquid first, then softer ingredients and harder items like ice or frozen fruit last.

(It helps a lot to blend fruits with liquid first before adding other ingredients. Check beginning of each section for special instructions)

2. Blend on medium and increase to high for 1 minute. Repeat as necessary.

VANILLA BEAN CASHEW MILK

Ingredients

1 cup soaked unsalted organic cashews
4 cups filtered or purified water
pinch of himalayan sea salt
1 tbsp local raw honey or other sweetener
1 vanilla bean

Directions:

1. Add liquid first, then softer ingredients and harder items like ice or frozen fruit last.

(It helps a lot to blend fruits with liquid first before adding other ingredients. Check beginning of each section for special instructions)

2. Blend on medium and increase to high for 1 minute. Repeat as necessary.

HOMEMADE MACADAMIA NUT MILK

Ingredients

½ cup organic, soaked macadamia nuts
3½ cups cold water
4 Medjool dates, pitted
½ teaspoon vanilla extract

Directions:

1. Add liquid first, then softer ingredients and harder items like ice or frozen fruit last.

(It helps a lot to blend fruits with liquid first before adding other ingredients. Check beginning of each section for special instructions)

2. Blend on medium and increase to high for 1 minute. Repeat as necessary.

DECADENT ALMOND MACADAMIA MILK

Ingredients

50g macadamia
150g almond
30g dates
1 l of water

Directions:

1. Add liquid first, then softer ingredients and harder items like ice or frozen fruit last.

(It helps a lot to blend fruits with liquid first before adding other ingredients. Check beginning of each section for special instructions)

2. Blend on medium and increase to high for 1 minute. Repeat as necessary.

HOMEMADE ALMOND MACADAMIA ICED COFFEE

Ingredients
½ cup blanched almonds
¼ cup soaked macadamia nuts
6 pitted dates
2½ cups water

Directions:
1. Add liquid first, then softer ingredients and harder items like ice or frozen fruit last.

(It helps a lot to blend fruits with liquid first before adding other ingredients. Check beginning of each section for special instructions)

2. Blend on medium and increase to high for 1 minute. Repeat as necessary.

WALNUT COCONUT MILK WITH TURMERIC AND CINNAMON

Ingredients
1 cup soaked walnuts.
1 cup shredded coconut
1 tsp. Vanilla Extract
1 tsp. Cinnamon
1 tsp. Turmeric
1 tsp. Honey
a pinch of pink Himalayan salt
4 cups of water

Directions:
1. Add liquid first, then softer ingredients and harder items like ice or frozen fruit last.

(It helps a lot to blend fruits with liquid first before adding other ingredients. Check beginning of each section for special instructions)

2. Blend on medium and increase to high for 1 minute. Repeat as necessary.

BANANA ALMOND AND OAT SMOOTHIE - ZUPAS

Ingredients
1 cup almond milk
1 tbsp natural peanut butter
1/4 cup soaked whole almonds
1/4 cup ground flax seed
1 cup plain Greek yogurt
1 tbsp honey
1/2 cup raw old fashioned oatmeal
2-3 bananas (best if cut into chunks and frozen)
1 tsp vanilla
1-2 dried dates (optional, to help sweeten)
2 cups crushed ice

Directions:
1. Add liquid first, then softer ingredients and harder items like ice or frozen fruit last.

(It helps a lot to blend fruits with liquid first before adding other ingredients. Check beginning of each section for special instructions)

2. Blend on medium and increase to high for 1 minute. Repeat as necessary.

VANILLA WALNUT MILK

Ingredients
5 cups water
1 cup soaked walnuts
1 tbsps agave nectar
1 tbsp vanilla extract
1/4 teaspoon sea salt

Directions:
1. Add liquid first, then softer ingredients and harder items like ice or frozen fruit last.

(It helps a lot to blend fruits with liquid first before adding other ingredients. Check beginning of each section for special instructions)
2. Blend on medium and increase to high for 1 minute. Repeat as necessary.

PUMPKIN SPICE ALMOND MILK

Ingredients
1 cup soaked organic almonds (soaked overnight)
2 teaspoons vanilla extract or 1 vanilla bean (soaked with the almonds)
4 cups filtered water
1/2 cup organic pumpkin purée (canned or fresh)
2 teaspoons ground cinnamon
1/4 teaspoon ground nutmeg
pinch of ground ginger
pinch of ground cloves
2 tbsps honey or maple syrup or a couple of soft medjool dates*
pinch of sea salt
Directions:
1. Add liquid first, then softer ingredients and harder items like ice or frozen fruit last.
(It helps a lot to blend fruits with liquid first before adding other ingredients. Check beginning of each section for special instructions)
2. Blend on medium and increase to high for 1 minute. Repeat as necessary.

ICED ALMOND-MACADAMIA MILK LATTE

Ingredients
1 generous cup/150 grams blanched almonds
1/2 cup/50 grams macadamia nuts
1/3 cup/40 grams pitted dates
1 liter filtered water
Directions:

1. Add liquid first, then softer ingredients and harder items like ice or frozen fruit last.
(It helps a lot to blend fruits with liquid first before adding other ingredients. Check beginning of each section for special instructions)
2. Blend on medium and increase to high for 1 minute. Repeat as necessary.

CHESTNUT PRALINE LATTE

Ingredients
1 cup (8 ounces) hot strong coffee
½ cup unsweetened cashew milk or other non-dairy milk, heated
3 roasted chestnuts (~ 1½ tablespoons)
6 toasted pecans (~ 1½ tablespoons)
2 tablespoons organic coconut sugar
½ teaspoon vanilla extract
Directions:
1. Add liquid first, then softer ingredients and harder items like ice or frozen fruit last.
(It helps a lot to blend fruits with liquid first before adding other ingredients. Check beginning of each section for special instructions)
2. Blend on medium and increase to high for 1 minute. Repeat as necessary.

ORANGE SPLASH PISTACHIO MILK

½ cup soaked unsalted pistachio nuts
2 Tablespoons honey
¼ teaspoon ground vanilla or ½ teaspoon vanilla extract
1/8 teaspoon ground cardamom
2 pinches sea salt
1 teaspoon orange blossom water, more to taste
Directions:
1. Add liquid first, then softer ingredients and harder items like ice or frozen fruit last.

(It helps a lot to blend fruits with liquid
first before adding other ingredients.
Check beginning of each section for
special instructions)
  2. Blend on medium and increase to
high for 1 minute. Repeat as necessary.

10 NUT BUTTER RECIPES

Directions:
1. Blend the nuts into a flour-like consistency first. Use the milling blade.
2. Add in rest of the ingredients according to the recipe.
3. Blend for 30-60 seconds. Repeat as necessary.

HOMEMADE ALMOND BUTTER

Ingredients
3 cups raw unsalted almonds
2 tbsps of coconut oil
dash of sea salt
Optional add ins:
1 tbsp of honey
1 tbsp of cinnamon
Directions:
1. Blend the nuts into a flour-like consistency first. Use the milling blade.
2. Add in rest of the ingredients according to the recipe.
3. Blend for 30-60 seconds. Repeat as necessary.

PECAN BUTTER

Ingredients
8 ounces (about two cups) high quality pecans, either whole or in pieces
sea salt, to taste
dash of cinnamon
Directions:
1. Blend the nuts into a flour-like consistency first. Use the milling blade.
2. Add in rest of the ingredients according to the recipe.
3. Blend for 30-60 seconds. Repeat as necessary.

WALNUT BUTTER

Ingredients
2 cups walnuts, shelled

¼ teaspoon salt
1 teaspoon honey
1 teaspoon roasted cinnamon
2 teaspoons walnut oil or grapeseed or canola oil
Directions:
1. Blend the nuts into a flour-like consistency first. Use the milling blade.
2. Add in rest of the ingredients according to the recipe.
3. Blend for 30-60 seconds. Repeat as necessary.

CHOCOLATE HAZELNUT BUTTER SPREAD

Ingredients
18 ounces hazelnuts
3 tbsp – ¼ cup cocoa powder
¼ – ½ cup coconut sugar or granulated sugar
⅛ teaspoon salt
Directions:
1. Blend the nuts into a flour-like consistency first. Use the milling blade.
2. Add in rest of the ingredients according to the recipe.
3. Blend for 30-60 seconds. Repeat as necessary.

CASHEW BUTTER

Ingredients
2 cups roasted cashews
2 tbsps organic coconut oil
1 tbsp pure vanilla extract
1/2 teaspoon sea salt
Directions:
1. Blend the nuts into a flour-like consistency first. Use the milling blade.
2. Add in rest of the ingredients according to the recipe.
3. Blend for 30-60 seconds. Repeat as necessary.

PISTACHIO BUTTER

Ingredients

2 cups roasted pistachios
1/4 tsp kosher salt
1 tbsp honey
1/8 tsp cinnamon
Directions:
1.   Blend the nuts into a flour-like consistency first. Use the milling blade.
2.   Add in rest of the ingredients according to the recipe.
3.   Blend for 30-60 seconds. Repeat as necessary.

PINE NUT BUTTER

Ingredients
2 cups of pine nuts
1 tbsp canola oil
1/4 teaspoon fine grain sea salt
Directions:
1.   Blend the nuts into a flour-like consistency first. Use the milling blade.
2.   Add in rest of the ingredients according to the recipe.
3.   Blend for 30-60 seconds. Repeat as necessary.

MACADAMIA NUT BUTTER

Ingredients
1 pound macadamia nuts*
6 tbsps coconut oil
pinch of salt
4-6 tbsps raw honey (optional)
Directions:
1.   Blend the nuts into a flour-like consistency first. Use the milling blade.
2.   Add in rest of the ingredients according to the recipe.
3.   Blend for 30-60 seconds. Repeat as necessary.

BRAZIL NUT BUTTER

Ingredients
2 cups organic raw brazil nuts
OPTIONAL ADDITIONS
Salt
Stevia, honey or maple syrup
Vanilla or almond extract

Raw cocoa powder or cacao nibs
Puree of dried fruit
Directions:
1.   Blend the nuts into a flour-like consistency first. Use the milling blade.
2.   Add in rest of the ingredients according to the recipe.
3.   Blend for 30-60 seconds. Repeat as necessary.

HOMEMADE VANILLA CASHEW BUTTER

Ingredients
2 cups roasted cashews
2 tbsps organic coconut or vegetable oil
1 tbsp pure vanilla extract
1/2 teaspoon sea salt
Directions:
1.   Blend the nuts into a flour-like consistency first. Use the milling blade.
2.   Add in rest of the ingredients according to the recipe.
3.   Blend for 30-60 seconds. Repeat as necessary.

25 EASY SOUP RECIPES

Directions:
1. Add all the ingredients you wish to liquify to make the soup (liquids first, then soft ingredients)
2. Turn on machine and blend for up to 50 seconds.
3. Remove lid and add ingredients to add more textures to liquid soup (tomato chunks, croutons, veggies, etc.)
4. Re-blend for 1-5 seconds.

MINESTRONE SOUP

Ingredients
1 (15 oz) can white beans, drained and rinsed
32 oz container reduced sodium chicken broth (or vegetable broth)
2 tsp olive oil
1/2 cup chopped onion
1 cup diced carrots
1/2 cup diced celery
2 garlic cloves, minced
1 (28 oz) can petite diced tomatoes
Parmesan cheese rind (optional)
1 fresh rosemary sprig
2 bay leaves
2 tbsp chopped fresh basil
1/4 cup chopped fresh Italian parsley
1/2 tsp kosher salt and fresh black pepper
1 medium 8 oz zucchini, diced
2 cups chopped fresh (or frozen defrosted) spinach
2 cups cooked small pasta such as ditalini or elbows (al dente)
extra parmesan cheese for garnish (optional)

Directions:
1. Add all the ingredients you wish to liquify to make the soup (liquids first, then soft ingredients)
2. Turn on machine and blend for up to 50 seconds.

3. Remove lid and add ingredients to add more textures to liquid soup (tomato chunks, croutons, veggies, etc.)
4. Re-blend for 1-5 seconds.

HEARTY VEGETABLE SOUP

Ingredients
1 tbsp olive oil
1 teaspoon minced garlic
1 1/2 pound lean ground beef
1/2 cup chopped onion
2 small potatoes, peeled and diced
1 cup chopped celery
1 cup chopped carrots
1 (14.5 ounce) can rotel
1 (15 ounce) can tomato sauce
1 cup water
1 tbsp balsamic vinegar
2 teaspoons chili powder
1/2 teaspoon kosher salt
1/2 teaspoon ground black pepper
3 tomatoes, diced

Directions:
1. Add all the ingredients you wish to liquify to make the soup (liquids first, then soft ingredients)
2. Turn on machine and blend for up to 50 seconds.
3. Remove lid and add ingredients to add more textures to liquid soup (tomato chunks, croutons, veggies, etc.)
4. Re-blend for 1-5 seconds.

TURKEY MEATBALL SPINACH TORTELLINI SOUP

Ingredients
For the Meatballs:
10 oz 93% ground turkey
2 tbsp seasoned whole wheat breadcrumbs
2 tbsp grated parmesan cheese (Parmigiano Reggiano)
2 tbsp parsley, finely chopped
1 large egg
1 clove garlic, minced

1/8 tsp kosher salt
For the soup:
1/2 tbsp unsalted butter
2 stalks of celery, chopped
1 small onion, chopped
1 large carrot, peeled & chopped
2 cloves of garlic, minced
4 (14.5 oz) cans reduced sodium chicken broth
1 small Parmigiano-Reggiano rind (optional)
9 oz refrigerated spinach cheese tortellini
fresh ground black pepper, to taste
3 cups loosely packed baby spinach
fresh grated Parmigiano-Reggiano for topping
Directions:
1. Add all the ingredients you wish to liquify to make the soup (liquids first, then soft ingredients)
2. Turn on machine and blend for up to 50 seconds.
3. Remove lid and add ingredients to add more textures to liquid soup (tomato chunks, croutons, veggies, etc.)
4. Re-blend for 1-5 seconds.

CREAMY POTATO SOUP

Ingredients
1 (30 oz.) bag frozen hash-brown potatoes
2 (14 oz.) cans chicken broth
1 (10.75 oz.) can cream of chicken soup
½ cup chopped onion
¼ teaspoon ground black pepper (more to taste)
1 (8oz) package cream cheese (softened)
Optional Toppings: cheese, bacon, sliced green onions
Directions:
1. Add all the ingredients you wish to liquify to make the soup (liquids first, then soft ingredients)

2. Turn on machine and blend for up to 50 seconds.
3. Remove lid and add ingredients to add more textures to liquid soup (tomato chunks, croutons, veggies, etc.)
4. Re-blend for 1-5 seconds.

COPYCAT PANERA CREAMY TOMATO BASIL SOUP

Ingredients
1 28 oz can crushed tomatoes
1 28 oz can diced tomatoes
1 tbsp crushed garlic
1 14 oz can chicken broth {or 2 cups}
2 tbsp sugar
1/3 cup butter
1 cup heavy cream
15-20 basil leaves, chopped
Directions:
1. Add all the ingredients you wish to liquify to make the soup (liquids first, then soft ingredients)
2. Turn on machine and blend for up to 50 seconds.
3. Remove lid and add ingredients to add more textures to liquid soup (tomato chunks, croutons, veggies, etc.)
4. Re-blend for 1-5 seconds.

5 - INGREDIENT BROCCOLI CHEESE SOUP

Ingredients
4 cups chicken stock
2 cups cooked broccoli florets, chopped
½ small onion, diced
15 oz can evaporated milk
2 cups shredded sharp cheddar cheese
Salt and Pepper To Taste
Directions:
5. Add all the ingredients you wish to liquify to make the soup (liquids first, then soft ingredients)
6. Turn on machine and blend for up to 50 seconds.

7. Remove lid and add ingredients to add more textures to liquid soup (tomato chunks, croutons, veggies, etc.)
8. Re-blend for 1-5 seconds.

8 CAN TACO SOUP

Ingredients
1 (15 oz.) can black beans, drained and rinsed
1 (15 oz.) can pinto beans, drained and rinsed
1 (14.5 oz.) can petite diced tomatoes, drained
1 (15.25 oz.) can sweet corn, drained
1 (12.5 oz.) can white chicken breast, drained
1 (10.75 oz.) can cream of chicken soup
1 (10 oz.) can green enchilada sauce
1 (14 oz.) can chicken broth
1 packet taco seasoning
Directions:
1. Add all the ingredients you wish to liquify to make the soup (liquids first, then soft ingredients)
2. Turn on machine and blend for up to 50 seconds.
3. Remove lid and add ingredients to add more textures to liquid soup (tomato chunks, croutons, veggies, etc.)
4. Re-blend for 1-5 seconds.

ROASTED CAULIFLOWER AND BROCCOLI WHITE CHEDDAR SOUP

Ingredients
1 large head cauliflower, cut into florets
1 medium head broccoli, cut into florets
1 tablespoon olive oil
8 strips uncooked bacon
2 medium onions, chopped
1/2 head garlic, minced
8 cups chicken stock
1 cup heavy cream
8oz (about 2 cups) shredded white cheddar cheese

2 tablespoons fresh thyme leaves, roughly chopped
salt & pepper to taste
Directions:
1. Add all the ingredients you wish to liquify to make the soup (liquids first, then soft ingredients)
2. Turn on machine and blend for up to 50 seconds.
3. Remove lid and add ingredients to add more textures to liquid soup (tomato chunks, croutons, veggies, etc.)
4. Re-blend for 1-5 seconds.

SAUSAGE, POTATO AND SPINACH SOUP

Ingredients
1 tbsp olive oil
1 pound spicy Italian sausage, casing removed
3 cloves garlic, minced
1 onion, diced
1/2 teaspoon dried oregano
1/2 teaspoon dried basil
1/2 teaspoon crushed red pepper flakes, optional
Kosher salt and freshly ground black pepper, to taste
5 cups chicken broth
1 bay leaf
1 pound red potatoes, diced
3 cups baby spinach
1/4 cup heavy cream
Directions:
1. Add all the ingredients you wish to liquify to make the soup (liquids first, then soft ingredients)
2. Turn on machine and blend for up to 50 seconds.
3. Remove lid and add ingredients to add more textures to liquid soup (tomato chunks, croutons, veggies, etc.)
4. Re-blend for 1-5 seconds.

CREAMY CHICKEN AND MUSHROOM SOUP

Ingredients
1 tbsp olive oil
8 ounces boneless, skinless chicken thighs, cut into 1-inch chunks
Kosher salt and freshly ground black pepper
2 tbsps unsalted butter
3 cloves garlic, minced
8 ounces cremini mushrooms, thinly sliced
1 onion, diced
3 carrots, peeled and diced
2 stalks celery, diced
1/2 teaspoon dried thyme
1/4 cup all-purpose flour
4 cups chicken stock
1 bay leaf
1/2 cup half and half, or more, as needed*
2 tbsps chopped fresh parsley leaves
1 sprig rosemary
Directions:
1.   Add all the ingredients you wish to liquify to make the soup (liquids first, then soft ingredients)
2.   Turn on machine and blend for up to 50 seconds.
3.   Remove lid and add ingredients to add more textures to liquid soup (tomato chunks, croutons, veggies, etc.)
4.   Re-blend for 1-5 seconds.

BEST EVER MUSHROOM SOUP

Ingredients
1 large white onion, diced
1 package white button mushrooms (10 oz) sliced
1 package baby portobello mushrooms (10 oz) sliced
10 stalks fresh thyme, leaves removed
1 cup organic vegetable broth

1 tbs. tapioca flour
1 cup almond or cashew milk (unsweetened)
1 dried bay leaf
½ tbs. liquid aminos (GF) (or soy sauce)
½ tsp. salt
freshly ground pepper
Directions:
1.   Add all the ingredients you wish to liquify to make the soup (liquids first, then soft ingredients)
2.   Turn on machine and blend for up to 50 seconds.
3.   Remove lid and add ingredients to add more textures to liquid soup (tomato chunks, croutons, veggies, etc.)
4.   Re-blend for 1-5 seconds.

QUICK AND EASY TOMATO SOUP

Ingredients
3 tbsps olive oil
2 tbsps butter
1 large sweet onion, finely chopped
2 large cloves garlic, minced
2 tbsps all-purpose flour
2 teaspoons dried basil
2 teaspoons dried thyme
4 cups chicken broth
56 ounces canned crushed tomatoes
2 teaspoons sugar
½ teaspoon kosher salt
½ teaspoon ground black pepper
optional garnish: chopped fresh basil, chives, or dill
Directions:
1.   Add all the ingredients you wish to liquify to make the soup (liquids first, then soft ingredients)
2.   Turn on machine and blend for up to 50 seconds.
3.   Remove lid and add ingredients to add more textures to liquid soup (tomato chunks, croutons, veggies, etc.)
4.   Re-blend for 1-5 seconds.

EASY CHICKEN AND RICE SOUP

Ingredients

1 tbsp extra-virgin olive oil
½ medium onion, chopped
½ garlic cloves, minced
1 medium carrot, cut diagonally into 1/2-inch-thick slices
1 celery ribs, halved lengthwise, and cut into 1/2-inch-thick slices
2 fresh thyme sprigs
1 bay leaf
2 cups chicken stock or broth (we use low sodium)
1 cup of water
½ cup long grain white rice (cooked)
½ cup shredded cooked chicken breasts
Kosher salt and freshly ground black pepper

Directions:

1. Add all the ingredients you wish to liquify to make the soup (liquids first, then soft ingredients)
2. Turn on machine and blend for up to 50 seconds.
3. Remove lid and add ingredients to add more textures to liquid soup (tomato chunks, croutons, veggies, etc.)
4. Re-blend for 1-5 seconds.

QUICK & EASY CHINESE NOODLE SOUP

Ingredients

4 cups/1 Litre chicken Stock
2 – 3 Green/Spring onions – finely sliced into rounds
1 tbsp Oyster Sauce
1 tbsp Light Soy Sauce
1 tbsp Dark Soy Sauce
4 oz/200g Dried Chinese noodles
4 Bok Choy/Pak choi leaves, sliced

Directions:

1. Add all the ingredients you wish to liquify to make the soup (liquids first, then soft ingredients)
2. Turn on machine and blend for up to 50 seconds.
3. Remove lid and add ingredients to add more textures to liquid soup (tomato chunks, croutons, veggies, etc.)
4. Re-blend for 1-5 seconds.

OLIVE GARDEN'S HOMEMADE ZUPPA TOSCANA SOUP

Ingredients

5-7 slices of cooked bacon
1/2 lb hot Italian Sausage
5 medium russet potatoes, washed and thinly sliced
2 cups kale, chopped
1 cups heavy whipping cream
1 quart water
2 cans chicken broth
1/2 large onion, finely chopped
4 medium cloves of garlic, minced
2 teaspoon red pepper flakes
salt and pepper
grated Parmesan for sprinkling

Directions:

1. Add all the ingredients you wish to liquify to make the soup (liquids first, then soft ingredients)
2. Turn on machine and blend for up to 50 seconds.
3. Remove lid and add ingredients to add more textures to liquid soup (tomato chunks, croutons, veggies, etc.)
4. Re-blend for 1-5 seconds.

EASY CHEESEBURGER SOUP

Ingredients

1 pound ground beef, cooked
1 cup diced carrots
1/2 cup diced celery
1/2 onion, diced
1 tbsp butter

4 cups chicken broth
1 teaspoon dried parsley
1 cup Velveeta cheese, cubed
1 cup milk
salt and pepper to taste
Directions:
1.   Add all the ingredients you wish to liquify to make the soup (liquids first, then soft ingredients)
2.   Turn on machine and blend for up to 50 seconds.
3.   Remove lid and add ingredients to add more textures to liquid soup (tomato chunks, croutons, veggies, etc.)
4.   Re-blend for 1-5 seconds.

BEST BUTTERNUT SQUASH SOUP

Ingredients
2 large roasted butternut squashes
1 pint of half and half
¾ stick of butter (browned)
2 tbsp of oil
Salt and pepper to taste
2½ cups of chicken stock
Creme fraiche to garnish
Directions:
1.   Add all the ingredients you wish to liquify to make the soup (liquids first, then soft ingredients)
2.   Turn on machine and blend for up to 50 seconds.
3.   Remove lid and add ingredients to add more textures to liquid soup (tomato chunks, croutons, veggies, etc.)
4.   Re-blend for 1-5 seconds.

MISO SOUP

Ingredients
1 quart vegetable or chicken stock
2 cups water
2 to 3 tbsps Miso paste
1/3 of a 14 oz block of firm tofu, cut in small cubes

2 cups assorted mushrooms, sliced or left whole if very small
4 or 5 scallions, sliced thin (use all of the white and a little of the green)
Directions:
1.   Add all the ingredients you wish to liquify to make the soup (liquids first, then soft ingredients)
2.   Turn on machine and blend for up to 50 seconds.
3.   Remove lid and add ingredients to add more textures to liquid soup (tomato chunks, croutons, veggies, etc.)
4.   Re-blend for 1-5 seconds.

MEXICAN LIME SOUP W/ CHICKEN

Ingredients
3 or 4 limes
3 bone-in, chicken breast halves
1 tsp salt
1/2 tsp ground pepper
1 Tbs olive oil
1 large white onion, chopped
5 garlic cloves, minced
8 oz diced green chilies
4 cups low-sodium chicken broth
4 cups water
1 1/2 tsp. ground cumin
1 avocado, peeled (sliced or chopped)
Shredded Monterrey jack cheese
Directions:
1.   Add all the ingredients you wish to liquify to make the soup (liquids first, then soft ingredients)
2.   Turn on machine and blend for up to 50 seconds.
3.   Remove lid and add ingredients to add more textures to liquid soup (tomato chunks, croutons, veggies, etc.)
4.   Re-blend for 1-5 seconds.

CREAMY SWEET POTATO SOUP

Ingredients

2 tbsps olive oil
1 small onion, diced
1 shallot, diced
2 cloves garlic, chopped
3-4 medium sized sweet potatoes (about 2 pounds), peeled cut into 1-inch cubes
4 cups chicken (or vegetable) stock
1/2 teaspoon cinnamon
1 teaspoon paprika
1 -2 teaspoons salt
Fresh ground pepper
Directions:
1. Add all the ingredients you wish to liquify to make the soup (liquids first, then soft ingredients)
2. Turn on machine and blend for up to 50 seconds.
3. Remove lid and add ingredients to add more textures to liquid soup (tomato chunks, croutons, veggies, etc.)
4. Re-blend for 1-5 seconds.

EASY CHICKEN NOODLE SOUP

Ingredients
4 cups water
1 can (14-1/2 ounces) chicken broth
1-1/2 cups cubed cooked chicken breast
1 can (10-3/4 ounces) condensed cream of chicken soup, undiluted
3/4 cup sliced celery
3/4 cup sliced carrots
1 small onion, chopped
1-1/2 teaspoons dried parsley flakes
1 teaspoon reduced-sodium chicken bouillon granules
1/4 teaspoon pepper
3 cups cooked egg noodles
Directions:
1. Add all the ingredients you wish to liquify to make the soup (liquids first, then soft ingredients)

2. Turn on machine and blend for up to 50 seconds.
3. Remove lid and add ingredients to add more textures to liquid soup (tomato chunks, croutons, veggies, etc.)
4. Re-blend for 1-5 seconds.

CHICKEN ENCHILADA SOUP

Ingredients
1st Blend:
3 Roma or other small tomatoes
1 carrot
3 to 4 sweet peppers
1 celery stalk
1/2 cup mushrooms
4 sprigs cilantro
1 tablespoon taco seasoning
1 tablespoon tomato bouillon**
1/2 teaspoon garlic salt
3 cups water*
2nd Blend:
1 cup black beans (drained)
1 cup corn (drained)
1 cup cooked chicken, shredded or cubed
1 cup tortilla chips
Directions:
1. Add all the ingredients you wish to liquify to make the soup (liquids first, then soft ingredients)
2. Turn on machine and blend for up to 50 seconds.
3. Remove lid and add ingredients to add more textures to liquid soup (tomato chunks, croutons, veggies, etc.)
4. Re-blend for 1-5 seconds.

5-INGREDIENT EASY WHITE CHICKEN CHILI

Ingredients
6 cups chicken broth
4 cups cooked shredded chicken
2 (15-oz) cans beans, drained
2 cups salsa verde (store-bought or homemade

2 tsp. ground cumin
optional toppings: diced avocado, chopped fresh cilantro, shredded cheese, chopped green onions, sour cream, crumbled tortilla chips
2 tbsps olive oil
5 cloves of garlic
4 cups of chicken stock
2 teaspoons hot sauce
½ teaspoon salt
½ teaspoon pepper
¼ cup sour cream
1 teaspoon dried oregano
2 large carrots, sliced diagonally
2 celery ribs, cut in half lengthwise
2-3 garlic cloves, minced
1 bay leaf
1 1/2 teaspoons dried thyme
8 cups chicken broth
2/3 cups cooked quinoa
1 1/2 cups shredded chicken
salt and pepper

Directions:
1. Add all the ingredients you wish to liquify to make the soup (liquids first, then soft ingredients)
2. Turn on machine and blend for up to 50 seconds.
3. Remove lid and add ingredients to add more textures to liquid soup (tomato chunks, croutons, veggies, etc.)
4. Re-blend for 1-5 seconds.

BBQ CIRCUIT RUB

2 tbsps chili powder
1 tbsp kosher salt
1 tbsp paprika (for more kick, use hot paprika)
1 teaspoon onion powder
1 teaspoon garlic powder
1 teaspoon sugar
1/2 teaspoon cumin
1/2 teaspoon cayenne pepper
Directions:

1. Add all the ingredients you grind into a powder. Use the milling blade for best results.
2. Turn on machine and blend for up to 45 seconds.
3. Remove lid and check to see that only a fine powder remains. Re-blend for 1-5 seconds, as needed.

CAJUN SPICE MIX

Ingredients
1 teaspoon coarse salt
1 teaspoon ground black pepper
1 teaspoon onion powder
1 teaspoon cayenne pepper
1 teaspoon dried oregano
1 teaspoon dried thyme
2 teaspoons paprika
2 teaspoons garlic powder
Directions:
1. Add all the ingredients you grind into a powder. Use the milling blade for best results.
2. Turn on machine and blend for up to 45 seconds.
3. Remove lid and check to see that only a fine powder remains. Re-blend for 1-5 seconds, as needed.

CHILI AND TACO SEASONING
Ingredients
4 tbsps of chili powder
1 teaspoon garlic powder
1 teaspoon onion powder
1 teaspoon crushed red pepper flakes
1/4 teaspoon cayenne pepper
1 teaspoon dried oregano
2 teaspoons paprika
2 tbsps ground cumin
3 teaspoons sea salt
4 teaspoons black pepper
Directions:
1. Add all the ingredients you grind into a powder. Use the milling blade for best results.

2. Turn on machine and blend for up to 45 seconds.
3. Remove lid and check to see that only a fine powder remains. Re-blend for 1-5 seconds, as needed.

CREOLE SEASONING BLEND

Ingredients
½ teaspoons black pepper, freshly ground
½ teaspoons white pepper
⅔ teaspoons cayenne pepper
1 teaspoon salt
2 teaspoons garlic powder
2 teaspoons onion powder
2 teaspoons oregano
2 teaspoons paprika
1 teaspoon thyme
1 teaspoon basil
Directions:
1. Add all the ingredients you grind into a powder. Use the milling blade for best results.
2. Turn on machine and blend for up to 45 seconds.
3. Remove lid and check to see that only a fine powder remains. Re-blend for 1-5 seconds, as needed.

GREEK SEASONING

Ingredients
3 tbsps sweet paprika-
1/2 teaspoon Sea salt-
1/2 teaspoon Chopped onion
1/2 teaspoon Coriander seed
1/2 teaspoon Garlic salt
1/2 teaspoon Black peppercorns
1/2 teaspoon Turmeric
1/4 teaspoon Minced garlic
1/4 teaspoon Crushed red pepper
1/4 teaspoon Dark chili powder
1/4 teaspoon Mediterranean oregano
1/4 teaspoon Sage
Directions:

1. Add all the ingredients you grind into a powder. Use the milling blade for best results.
2. Turn on machine and blend for up to 45 seconds.
3. Remove lid and check to see that only a fine powder remains. Re-blend for 1-5 seconds, as needed.

GREEK SEASONING FOR CHICKEN GYROS

Ingredients
2 teaspoons salt
2 teaspoons dried oregano
1 1/2 teaspoons onion powder
2 teaspoons garlic powder
1 teaspoon cornstarch
1 teaspoon pepper
1 teaspoon dried parsley flakes
1/2 teaspoon ground cinnamon
1/2 teaspoon grated nutmeg
Directions:
1. Add all the ingredients you grind into a powder. Use the milling blade for best results.
2. Turn on machine and blend for up to 45 seconds.
3. Remove lid and check to see that only a fine powder remains. Re-blend for 1-5 seconds, as needed.

MONTREAL STEAK SEASONING

Ingredients
4 tbsps salt
1 tbsp black peppercorns
1 tbsp dehydrated onion
1/2 tbsp dehydrated garlic
1/2 tbsp crushed red pepper flakes
1 tbsp dried thyme leaves
1 tbsp dried rosemary leaves
2 teaspoons fennel seed
Directions:

1. Add all the ingredients you grind into a powder. Use the milling blade for best results.
2. Turn on machine and blend for up to 45 seconds.
3. Remove lid and check to see that only a fine powder remains. Re-blend for 1-5 seconds, as needed.

OLD BAY SEASONING

Ingredients
1 tbsp paprika
1 tbsp ground bay leaves
1/2 tbsp celery salt
1 tsp black pepper
1/2 tsp red pepper flakes
1/2 tsp white pepper
1/2 tsp all-spice
Directions:
1. Add all the ingredients you grind into a powder. Use the milling blade for best results.
2. Turn on machine and blend for up to 45 seconds.
3. Remove lid and check to see that only a fine powder remains. Re-blend for 1-5 seconds, as needed.

PICKLING SPICE RECIPE

Ingredients
6 tbsp Mustard Seed
3 tbsp Whole Allspice
6 tsp coriander seed
6 whole cloves
3 tsp ground ginger
3 tsp red pepper flakes
3 bay leaves
3 cinnamon sticks
Directions:
1. Add all the ingredients you grind into a powder. Use the milling blade for best results.
2. Turn on machine and blend for up to 45 seconds.

3. Remove lid and check to see that only a fine powder remains. Re-blend for 1-5 seconds, as needed.

POULTRY SEASONING

Ingredients
1 tbsp. rosemary
1 tbsp. oregano
2 tsp. sage
1 tbsp. ginger
1 tbsp. marjoram
1 tbsp. thyme
1 tsp. freshly ground black pepper
Directions:
1. Add all the ingredients you grind into a powder. Use the milling blade for best results.
2. Turn on machine and blend for up to 45 seconds.
3. Remove lid and check to see that only a fine powder remains. Re-blend for 1-5 seconds, as needed.

STEAK FAJITA SPICE BLEND

Ingredients
3 tbsps cornstarch
2 tbsps chili powder
1 tbsp kosher salt
1 tbsp paprika
1 teaspoon onion powder
1 teaspoon garlic powder
1 teaspoon sugar
1/2 teaspoon cumin
1/2 teaspoon cayenne pepper
Directions:
1. Add all the ingredients you grind into a powder. Use the milling blade for best results.
2. Turn on machine and blend for up to 45 seconds.
3. Remove lid and check to see that only a fine powder remains. Re-blend for 1-5 seconds, as needed.

SPICY SWEET POTATO FRIES SPICE MIX

Ingredients
2 tbsp ground coriander
1 tbsp ground fennel
1 tbsp dried oregano
1 tbsp Aleppo Pepper
2 tbsp kosher salt
Directions:
1. Add all the ingredients you grind into a powder. Use the milling blade for best results.
2. Turn on machine and blend for up to 45 seconds.
3. Remove lid and check to see that only a fine powder remains. Re-blend for 1-5 seconds, as needed.

TACO SEASONING

Ingredients
2 TBSP Cumin
5 TBSP, 1 TSP Chili Powder
2 TSP Red Pepper Flakes
2 TSP Garlic Powder
2 TSP Onion Powder
1 TBSP, 1 TSP Paprika
2 TBSP, 2 TSP kosher salt
1 TBSP, 1 TSP black pepper
Directions:
1. Add all the ingredients you grind into a powder. Use the milling blade for best results.
2. Turn on machine and blend for up to 45 seconds.
3. Remove lid and check to see that only a fine powder remains. Re-blend for 1-5 seconds, as needed.

ZIPPY LEMON PEPPER RUB

Ingredients
½ teaspoons Black Pepper, Freshly Ground
½ teaspoons White Pepper
⅔ teaspoons Cayenne Pepper
1 teaspoon Salt

2 teaspoons Garlic Powder
2 teaspoons Onion Powder
2 teaspoons Oregano
2 teaspoons Paprika
1 teaspoon Thyme
1 teaspoon Basil
Directions:
1. Add all the ingredients you grind into a powder. Use the milling blade for best results.
2. Turn on machine and blend for up to 45 seconds.
3. Remove lid and check to see that only a fine powder remains. Re-blend for 1-5 seconds, as needed.

ADOBO SEASONING

Ingredients
6 tbsps table salt
6 tbsps garlic powder
3 tbsps onion powder
3 tbsps ground black pepper
3 tbsps dried crushed Mexican oregano
3 tbsps ground cumin
3 tbsps anchiote seed seasoning

1-1/2 tbsps ground ancho chili powder
1-1/2 tbsps smoked paprika
1-1/2 tbsps ground turmeric
1-1/2 tbsps ground coriander
Directions:
1. Add all the ingredients you grind into a powder. Use the milling blade for best results.
2. Turn on machine and blend for up to 45 seconds.
3. Remove lid and check to see that only a fine powder remains. Re-blend for 1-5 seconds, as needed.

BASIC CURRY POWDER

Ingredients
2 dried red chiles, stemmed
1 tbsp coriander seeds
1 tbsp fennel seeds

1 teaspoon cumin seeds
1 teaspoon ground mace
1 teaspoon ground white pepper
1/2 teaspoon turmeric
Directions:
1. Add all the ingredients you grind into a powder. Use the milling blade for best results.
2. Turn on machine and blend for up to 45 seconds.
3. Remove lid and check to see that only a fine powder remains. Re-blend for 1-5 seconds, as needed.

CHINESE 5 SPICE BLEND

Ingredients
2 tbsps black peppercorns
2 tbsps whole cloves
3 cinnamon sticks, about 2-inches long
2 tbsps fennel seed
10 whole star anise
Directions:
1. Add all the ingredients you grind into a powder. Use the milling blade for best results.
2. Turn on machine and blend for up to 45 seconds.
3. Remove lid and check to see that only a fine powder remains. Re-blend for 1-5 seconds, as needed.

EGYPTIAN DUKKAH

Ingredients
1 cup nuts
1/2 cup sesame seeds
1/2 cup coriander seeds
1/4 cup cumin seeds
1 teaspoon sea salt
Freshly ground black pepper
Directions:
1. Add all the ingredients you grind into a powder. Use the milling blade for best results.
2. Turn on machine and blend for up to 45 seconds.

3. Remove lid and check to see that only a fine powder remains. Re-blend for 1-5 seconds, as needed.

ETHIOPIAN BERBERE

Ingredients
1 teaspoon ginger
1/4 teaspoon cinnamon
1/2 teaspoon cardamom
1/4 teaspoon allspice
1/2 teaspoon coriander
1/2 teaspoon cumin
1/2 teaspoon fenugreek
1/2 teaspoon nutmeg
1/4 teaspoon cloves
2 tbsps salt
1/4 cup paprika
1/2 cup cayenne pepper
Directions:
1. Add all the ingredients you grind into a powder. Use the milling blade for best results.
2. Turn on machine and blend for up to 45 seconds.
3. Remove lid and check to see that only a fine powder remains. Re-blend for 1-5 seconds, as needed.

GARAM MASALA

Ingredients
1 heaping teaspoon whole cloves
1 ½ teaspoon black cardamom seeds (about 10 whole pods)
6 heaping tbsps cumin seed
1 tbsp pounded cinnamon sticks
¼ teaspoon ground mace
¼ teaspoon ground nutmeg
Directions:
1. Add all the ingredients you grind into a powder. Use the milling blade for best results.
2. Turn on machine and blend for up to 45 seconds.

3. Remove lid and check to see that only a fine powder remains. Re-blend for 1-5 seconds, as needed.

APPLE PIE SPICE BLEND

Ingredients
¼ cup ground cinnamon
2 teaspoons ground nutmeg
1 teaspoon ground allspice
1 teaspoon ground ginger
Directions:
1. Add all the ingredients you grind into a powder. Use the milling blade for best results.
2. Turn on machine and blend for up to 45 seconds.
3. Remove lid and check to see that only a fine powder remains. Re-blend for 1-5 seconds, as needed.

CHAI SPICE BLEND

Ingredients
2-4 cardamom pods (seeds only)
6-7 cloves
1 stick cassia cinnamon (1 cm x 4 cm in area), broken into tiny pieces
8-10 black peppercorns (smashed)
1 tbsp dried ginger powder
Directions:
1. Add all the ingredients you grind into a powder. Use the milling blade for best results.
2. Turn on machine and blend for up to 45 seconds.
3. Remove lid and check to see that only a fine powder remains. Re-blend for 1-5 seconds, as needed.

GINGERBREAD SPICE MIX

Ingredients
1 1/2 teaspoons coriander seed
9 blades mace
15 cardamom pods
6 star anise petals
24 allspice berries
1 1/2 teaspoons black peppercorns

6 teaspoons freshly ground ginger
1 1/2 teaspoons ground cloves
1 1/2 teaspoons ground cinnamon
3/4 teaspoon freshly grated nutmeg
Directions:
1. Add all the ingredients you grind into a powder. Use the milling blade for best results.
2. Turn on machine and blend for up to 45 seconds.
3. Remove lid and check to see that only a fine powder remains. Re-blend for 1-5 seconds, as needed.

YELLOW CURRY POWDER

Ingredients
2 tbsp whole coriander seeds
1 tbsp whole cumin seeds
2 tsp whole black peppercorns
1 1/2 tsp whole brown mustard seeds
1 1/2 tsp ground turmeric
1 tsp whole fenugreek seeds
3 hot dried red chilies, crumbled
3 whole cloves
Directions:
1. Add all the ingredients you grind into a powder. Use the milling blade for best results.
2. Turn on machine and blend for up to 45 seconds.
3. Remove lid and check to see that only a fine powder remains. Re-blend for 1-5 seconds, as needed.

ZA'ATAR SEASONING BLEND

Ingredients
2 tbsps dried thyme
2 tbsps dried sumac
2 tbsps sesame seeds, toasted or untoasted
Directions:
1. Add all the ingredients you grind into a powder. Use the milling blade for best results.

2. Turn on machine and blend for up to
45 seconds.
3. Remove lid and check to see that only
a fine powder remains. Re-blend for 1-5
seconds, as needed.

25 FLAVORED COFFEE & TEA BLENDS

Directions:
1.   When making hot drinks, use the more heat-resistant larger containers (40-64 oz)
2.   Add the dry ingredients with some warm liquid and blend for 10-30 seconds to reduce to powder.(Be sure to strain out tea leaves before adding to blender)
3.   Next, add more liquid as necessary and blend until desired consistency is reached.

SKINNY VANILLA FRAPPUCCINO

Ingredients
1 pkg. Starbucks Via (Breakfast Blend)
2 tbsp. sugar-free vanilla flavored coffee creamer, powdered
1/2 cup fat free milk
8-10 ice cubes
1 packet Truvia
Directions:
1.   When making hot drinks, use the more heat-resistant larger containers (40-64 oz)
2.   Add the dry ingredients with some warm liquid and blend for 10-30 seconds to reduce to powder.(Be sure to strain out tea leaves before adding to blender)
3.   Next, add more liquid as necessary and blend until desired consistency is reached.

CHAI TEA FAUXCCINO

Ingredients
12 chai tea ice cubes (see notes above)
2 cups milks of choice (raw, almond or coconut)

2 tbsp maple syrup or raw honey (optional)
whipped cream (optional)
chocolate syrup (optional)
salted caramel sauce (optional)
Directions:
1.   When making hot drinks, use the more heat-resistant larger containers (40-64 oz)
2.   Add the dry ingredients with some warm liquid and blend for 10-30 seconds to reduce to powder.(Be sure to strain out tea leaves before adding to blender)
3.   Next, add more liquid as necessary and blend until desired consistency is reached.

PEPPERMINT MOCHA FRAPPE

Ingredients
4 oz_Coffee-mate peppermint mocha creamer
2 tbsp mocha cappuccino mix
3 cups ice cubes
whipped cream (optional)
sugar/chocolate sprinkles for topping
Directions:
1.   When making hot drinks, use the more heat-resistant larger containers (40-64 oz)
2.   Add the dry ingredients with some warm liquid and blend for 10-30 seconds to reduce to powder.(Be sure to strain out tea leaves before adding to blender)
3.   Next, add more liquid as necessary and blend until desired consistency is reached.

YOUTHBERRY WILD ORANGE BLOSSOM TEA BLEND

Ingredients
apple pieces,
white tea,

hibiscus flowers,
rose hip peels,
apple slices,
candied pineapple pieces
candied mango pieces
beetroot pieces,
citrus slices,
citrus peels,
red currants,
orange juice pieces,
orange petals,
rose petals,
açai fruit powder
Directions:
1.   When making hot drinks, use the more heat-resistant larger containers (40-64 oz)
2.   Add the dry ingredients with some warm liquid and blend for 10-30 seconds to reduce to powder.(Be sure to strain out tea leaves before adding to blender)
3.   Next, add more liquid as necessary and blend until desired consistency is reached.

STRAWBERRY LEMONADE HERBAL TEA

Ingredients
apple pieces,
rosehip peels,
apple slices,
strawberry slices,
strawberry pieces,
natural and artificial flavoring,
marigold petals,
citric acid
Directions:
1.   When making hot drinks, use the more heat-resistant larger containers (40-64 oz)
2.   Add the dry ingredients with some warm liquid and blend for 10-30 seconds to reduce to powder.(Be sure

to strain out tea leaves before adding to blender)
3.   Next, add more liquid as necessary and blend until desired consistency is reached.

CHOCOLATE CHIP COOKIE COFFEE CREAMER

Ingredients
1 can (14oz) sweetened condensed milk
1 1/2 cup milk
3 tbsp unsweetened cocoa powder
3 tbsp light brown sugar, packed
2 tsp vanilla extract
Directions:
1.   When making hot drinks, use the more heat-resistant larger containers (40-64 oz)
2.   Add the dry ingredients with some warm liquid and blend for 10-30 seconds to reduce to powder.(Be sure to strain out tea leaves before adding to blender)
3.   Next, add more liquid as necessary and blend until desired consistency is reached.

SKINNY ICE BLENDED MOCHA

Ingredients
about 1½ cups crushed ice
½ cup non-fat milk
⅓ cup mashed ripe bananas
1 teaspoon pure vanilla extract
1 tbsp cocoa powder
2 teaspoons instant espresso powder
2 teaspoons granulated sugar
Directions:
1.   When making hot drinks, use the more heat-resistant larger containers (40-64 oz)
2.   Add the dry ingredients with some warm liquid and blend for 10-30 seconds to reduce to powder.(Be sure

to strain out tea leaves before adding to blender)

3.   Next, add more liquid as necessary and blend until desired consistency is reached.

CHOCOLATE FUDGE SUNDAE ICED COFFEE

Ingredients
Donut Shop regular iced coffee K-cup
2 scoops vanilla ice cream
hot fudge sauce, slightly warmed
ice
whipped cream
Directions:
1.   When making hot drinks, use the more heat-resistant larger containers (40-64 oz)
2.   Add the dry ingredients with some warm liquid and blend for 10-30 seconds to reduce to powder.(Be sure to strain out tea leaves before adding to blender)
3.   Next, add more liquid as necessary and blend until desired consistency is reached.

GREEN TEA FRAPPE

Ingredients
1 cup non-fat milk
55 grams (about ½ cup) honeydew melon
¼ tsp. green tea powder
½ tsp. stevia
¼ tsp. vanilla extract
6 - 8 ice cubes
⅛ tsp. xanthan gum (optional)
Directions:
1.   When making hot drinks, use the more heat-resistant larger containers (40-64 oz)
2.   Add the dry ingredients with some warm liquid and blend for 10-30 seconds to reduce to powder.(Be sure

LAVENDER TEA

Ingredients
3 cups of hot water
1   handful of fresh lemon balm. (Substitute mints or a couple of tea bags.)
2 tbsps fresh or dried lavender flowers. Honey to sweeten. (Optional.)
Directions:
1.   When making hot drinks, use the more heat-resistant larger containers (40-64 oz)
2.   Add the dry ingredients with some warm liquid and blend for 10-30 seconds to reduce to powder.(Be sure to strain out tea leaves before adding to blender)
3.   Next, add more liquid as necessary and blend until desired consistency is reached.

JACK FROST TEA

Ingredients
1/4 cup dried peppermint leaves
1/4 cup dried spearmint leaves
1 teaspoon of tisane
8 oz boiling water
Directions:
1.   When making hot drinks, use the more heat-resistant larger containers (40-64 oz)
2.   Add the dry ingredients with some warm liquid and blend for 10-30 seconds to reduce to powder.(Be sure to strain out tea leaves before adding to blender)
3.   Next, add more liquid as necessary and blend until desired consistency is reached.

MAKE YOUR OWN TRANQUIL TEA BLEND

Ingredients
4 parts chamomile
2 parts lemon grass
2 parts rose petals
Directions:
1.   When making hot drinks, use the more heat-resistant larger containers (40-64 oz)
2.   Add the dry ingredients with some warm liquid and blend for 10-30 seconds to reduce to powder.(Be sure to strain out tea leaves before adding to blender)
3.   Next, add more liquid as necessary and blend until desired consistency is reached.

ROSY BLACK TEA

Ingredients
2 parts rose petals
1 part black tea
8 oz boiling water
Directions:
1.   When making hot drinks, use the more heat-resistant larger containers (40-64 oz)
2.   Add the dry ingredients with some warm liquid and blend for 10-30 seconds to reduce to powder.(Be sure to strain out tea leaves before adding to blender)
3.   Next, add more liquid as necessary and blend until desired consistency is reached.

NETTLE CINNAMON HERBAL TEA INFUSION

Ingredients
2 parts nettle
2 parts rose hips
1 part cinnamon chips
4 cups filtered water

Ice (optional)
Raw honey or fresh fruit juice (optional)
Directions:
1.   When making hot drinks, use the more heat-resistant larger containers (40-64 oz)
2.   Add the dry ingredients with some warm liquid and blend for 10-30 seconds to reduce to powder.(Be sure to strain out tea leaves before adding to blender)
3.   Next, add more liquid as necessary and blend until desired consistency is reached.

AFTER-DINNER DIGESTIVE TEA

Ingredients
3 ounces spearmint leaves
grams dried licorice root
Directions:
1.   When making hot drinks, use the more heat-resistant larger containers (40-64 oz)
2.   Add the dry ingredients with some warm liquid and blend for 10-30 seconds to reduce to powder.(Be sure to strain out tea leaves before adding to blender)
3.   Next, add more liquid as necessary and blend until desired consistency is reached.

APPLE GREEN TEA TURMERIC TONIC

Ingredients
4 parts nettle (Urtica dioica) leaf
3 parts spearmint (Mentha spicata) leaf
3 parts lemon balm (Melissa officinalis)
2 parts mullein (Verbascum thapsus) leaf
2 parts (combined) dandelion (Taraxacum officinale) leaf and root
2 parts red clover (Trifolium pratense) blossoms 1 part rose (Rosa spp.) hips

1 part Ginger Root (dried cut and sifted)
Directions:
1.   When making hot drinks, use the more heat-resistant larger containers (40-64 oz)
2.   Add the dry ingredients with some warm liquid and blend for 10-30 seconds to reduce to powder.(Be sure to strain out tea leaves before adding to blender)
3.   Next, add more liquid as necessary and blend until desired consistency is reached.

HOMEMADE BLACK APPLE TEA MIX

Ingredients
1 sweet organic apple
2 T lemon juice
2 t turbinado sugar
1/2 C loose leaf black tea
15 whole cloves
2 cinnamon sticks, broken (to break cinnamon sticks, place on towel and fold towel over. hit with heavy object several times)
Directions:
1.   When making hot drinks, use the more heat-resistant larger containers (40-64 oz)
2.   Add the dry ingredients with some warm liquid and blend for 10-30 seconds to reduce to powder.(Be sure to strain out tea leaves before adding to blender)
3.   Next, add more liquid as necessary and blend until desired consistency is reached.

RUSSIAN TEA (NO POWDERED MIX)

Ingredients
4 cups water
Juice of one lemon (approx 1/2 cup)
Juice of two oranges (approx 1 cup)

2 tbsps honey
1 4" cinnamon stick
1 teaspoon whole cloves
4 black tea bags
Directions:
1.   When making hot drinks, use the more heat-resistant larger containers (40-64 oz)
2.   Add the dry ingredients with some warm liquid and blend for 10-30 seconds to reduce to powder.(Be sure to strain out tea leaves before adding to blender)
3.   Next, add more liquid as necessary and blend until desired consistency is reached.

SCHISANDRA FIVE-FLAVORED TEA

Ingredients
2 tbsp Schisandra berries
2 tbsp Elderberries (optional)
6 small pieces of licorice root, broken into small pieces
5-6 inch knob of ginger peeled and coarsely chopped
A palmful or two of dried eleuthero
1-2 tbsp of dried green stevia leaves
1-2 cinnamon sticks, crushed
Directions:
1.   When making hot drinks, use the more heat-resistant larger containers (40-64 oz)
2.   Add the dry ingredients with some warm liquid and blend for 10-30 seconds to reduce to powder.(Be sure to strain out tea leaves before adding to blender)
3.   Next, add more liquid as necessary and blend until desired consistency is reached.

VITAMIN C HERBAL INFUSION

Ingredients

4 tbsps rose hips
1 tbsp lemongrass
1 tbsp cinnamon chips
1 teaspoon hibiscus flowers
1 teaspoon fennel seed
½ teaspoon lemon peel
4 cups filtered water
(optional)
Ice
Raw honey or fresh fruit juice
Directions:
1.   When making hot drinks, use the more heat-resistant larger containers (40-64 oz)
2.   Add the dry ingredients with some warm liquid and blend for 10-30 seconds to reduce to powder.(Be sure to strain out tea leaves before adding to blender)
3.   Next, add more liquid as necessary and blend until desired consistency is reached.

SKINNY MINT CHOCOLATE CHIP FRAPPUCINO

Ingredients
¾ c double-strength coffee, chilled
½ c skim milk
2 tbsp unsweetened cocoa powder
1/8 tsp peppermint extract
2 c ice cubes
sweetener, to taste (such as Stevia, Swerve, Truvia, etc.)
½ tsp miniature chocolate chips or dark chocolate, chopped
Directions:
1.   When making hot drinks, use the more heat-resistant larger containers (40-64 oz)
2.   Add the dry ingredients with some warm liquid and blend for 10-30 seconds to reduce to powder.(Be sure to strain out tea leaves before adding to blender)

3.   Next, add more liquid as necessary and blend until desired consistency is reached.

COCONUT WATER ICED COFFEE

Ingredients
1 cup coconut water
1/3-1/2 cup coffee concentrate
Optional: cream or coconut creme for stirring
Directions:
1.   When making hot drinks, use the more heat-resistant larger containers (40-64 oz)
2.   Add the dry ingredients with some warm liquid and blend for 10-30 seconds to reduce to powder.(Be sure to strain out tea leaves before adding to blender)
3.   Next, add more liquid as necessary and blend until desired consistency is reached.

FRENCH VANILLA COFFEE CREAMER

Ingredients
1 can (14oz) Fat free sweetened condensed milk
1 1/2 cup fat free milk (skim)
2 tsp vanilla extract
Directions:
1.   When making hot drinks, use the more heat-resistant larger containers (40-64 oz)
2.   Add the dry ingredients with some warm liquid and blend for 10-30 seconds to reduce to powder.(Be sure to strain out tea leaves before adding to blender)
3.   Next, add more liquid as necessary and blend until desired consistency is reached.

LEMON BALM TEA

Ingredients
2 tbsps dried lemon balm
1 tbsp dried oatstraw
2 teaspoons dried, seedless rosehips
1 1/2 teaspoons dried orange peel
1/2 teaspoon dried lavender
Directions:
1.   When making hot drinks, use the more heat-resistant larger containers (40-64 oz)
2.   Add the dry ingredients with some warm liquid and blend for 10-30 seconds to reduce to powder.(Be sure to strain out tea leaves before adding to blender)
3.   Next, add more liquid as necessary and blend until desired consistency is reached.

HOMEMADE CINNAMON COFFEE

Ingredients
10 cups of water
3 whole cinnamon sticks
3 heaping teaspoons brown sugar
1 cup ground coffee (unflavored)
1 teaspoon cinnamon
Directions:
1.   When making hot drinks, use the more heat-resistant larger containers (40-64 oz)
2.   Add the dry ingredients with some warm liquid and blend for 10-30 seconds to reduce to powder.(Be sure to strain out tea leaves before adding to blender)
3.   Next, add more liquid as necessary and blend until desired consistency is reached.

20 Milkshake Recipes

Directions:
1. Add soft ingredients and mix with liquid as per recipe.
2. Blend until desired consistency is achieved. Add more liquid to make less thicker shakes.
3. Open lid and add toppings to introduce more textures (crunchy candy pieces, soft fruit, etc.)
4. Blend for 5-10 seconds more if you want additional ingredients mixed in.

CAKE BATTER MILKSHAKE

Ingredients
2 cups vanilla ice cream
1 cup milk
1/2 cup vanilla or funfetti dry cake mix
Sprinkles (optional)

Directions:
1. Add soft ingredients and mix with liquid as per recipe.
2. Blend until desired consistency is achieved. Add more liquid to make less thicker shakes.
3. Open lid and add toppings to introduce more textures (crunchy candy pieces, soft fruit, etc.)
4. Blend for 5-10 seconds more if you want additional ingredients mixed in.

FROZEN CARAMEL HOT CHOCOLATE

Ingredients
2 cups prepared caramel hot chocolate
2 cups ice
¼ cup Caramel ice cream topping
1 cup Non-fat Cool Whip
¼ cup Rolos, chopped in half (optional)
¼ cup caramel chips (optional)
Directions:

1. Add soft ingredients and mix with liquid as per recipe.
2. Blend until desired consistency is achieved. Add more liquid to make less thicker shakes.
3. Open lid and add toppings to introduce more textures (crunchy candy pieces, soft fruit, etc.)
4. Blend for 5-10 seconds more if you want additional ingredients mixed in.

COOKIE MONSTER ICE CREAM

Ingredients
2 cup vanilla ice cream
14 oz sweetened <u>condensed milk</u>
1 tbsp vanilla extract (optional)
½ tsp blue food coloring
5 chocolate sandwich cookies (like Oreos)
2 chocolate chip cookies
Directions:
1. Add soft ingredients and mix with liquid as per recipe.
2. Blend until desired consistency is achieved. Add more liquid to make less thicker shakes.
3. Open lid and add toppings to introduce more textures (crunchy candy pieces, soft fruit, etc.)
4. Blend for 5-10 seconds more if you want additional ingredients mixed in.

STRAWBERRY NUTELLA MILKSHAKE

Ingredients
1/2 cup milk
1/2 cup strawberries
2 big scoops of vanilla ice cream
1/4 cup Nutella
Whipped cream, sprinkles, and extra Nutella, optional for serving
Directions:
1. Add soft ingredients and mix with liquid as per recipe.

2. Blend until desired consistency is achieved. Add more liquid to make less thicker shakes.
3. Open lid and add toppings to introduce more textures (crunchy candy pieces, soft fruit, etc.)
4. Blend for 5-10 seconds more if you want additional ingredients mixed in.

KIT KAT MILKSHAKE

Ingredients
1 Kit Kat bar (broken)
2 cups vanilla ice cream (or frozen yogurt)
1/2 cup milk
1 teaspoon vanilla extract
Hershey's chocolate syrup
Whipped cream
Directions:
1. Add soft ingredients and mix with liquid as per recipe.
2. Blend until desired consistency is achieved. Add more liquid to make less thicker shakes.
3. Open lid and add toppings to introduce more textures (crunchy candy pieces, soft fruit, etc.)
4. Blend for 5-10 seconds more if you want additional ingredients mixed in.

MINI S'MORE BROWNIE

Ingredients
1 box brownie mix
Mini graham cracker pie crusts
Mini marshmallows
Chocolate chips
Crushed graham crackers
Directions:
1. Add soft ingredients and mix with liquid as per recipe.
2. Blend until desired consistency is achieved. Add more liquid to make less thicker shakes.

3. Open lid and add toppings to introduce more textures (crunchy candy pieces, soft fruit, etc.)
4. Blend for 5-10 seconds more if you want additional ingredients mixed in.

NERDS MILKSHAKE

Ingredients
1st Blend:
3 scoops vanilla ice cream (or 1 heaping cup)
1/2 cup milk
2nd Blend:
one 1.65 ounce package strawberry & grape Nerds candy, extra if desired for garnish
whipped cream for topping if desired
Directions:
1. Add soft ingredients and mix with liquid as per recipe.
2. Blend until desired consistency is achieved. Add more liquid to make less thicker shakes.
3. Open lid and add toppings to introduce more textures (crunchy candy pieces, soft fruit, etc.)
4. Blend for 5-10 seconds more if you want additional ingredients mixed in.

SUPER EASY NUTELLA MILKSHAKE

Ingredients
2 scoops of Vanilla ice cream
4 Tbsp of Nutella (be generous!)
2 cups of milk
Directions:
1. Add soft ingredients and mix with liquid as per recipe.
2. Blend until desired consistency is achieved. Add more liquid to make less thicker shakes.
3. Open lid and add toppings to introduce more textures (crunchy candy pieces, soft fruit, etc.)

4. Blend for 5-10 seconds more if you want additional ingredients mixed in.

STRAWBERRY MILKSHAKE

Ingredients
1 cup milk
1 teaspoon vanilla
1 pound strawberries (hulled)
2 cups vanilla ice cream
Directions:
1. Add soft ingredients and mix with liquid as per recipe.
2. Blend until desired consistency is achieved. Add more liquid to make less thicker shakes.
3. Open lid and add toppings to introduce more textures (crunchy candy pieces, soft fruit, etc.)
4. Blend for 5-10 seconds more if you want additional ingredients mixed in.

COTTON CANDY MILKSHAKE

Ingredients
3 scoops of vanilla ice cream
2 tablespoons of milk
4 ice cubes
6 big puffs of cotton candy
Directions:
1. Add soft ingredients and mix with liquid as per recipe.
2. Blend until desired consistency is achieved. Add more liquid to make less thicker shakes.
3. Open lid and add toppings to introduce more textures (crunchy candy pieces, soft fruit, etc.)
4. Blend for 5-10 seconds more if you want additional ingredients mixed in.

BANANA CREAM PIE MILKSHAKE

Ingredients
1 cup Plain, Nonfat Greek Yogurt
¼ cup Unsweetened Vanilla Almond Milk
¼ tsp Vanilla Flavored Stevia Extract
1 medium Banana, very ripe
Crushed graham crackers
Directions:
1. Add soft ingredients and mix with liquid as per recipe.
2. Blend until desired consistency is achieved. Add more liquid to make less thicker shakes.
3. Open lid and add toppings to introduce more textures (crunchy candy pieces, soft fruit, etc.)
4. Blend for 5-10 seconds more if you want additional ingredients mixed in.

SNICKERS & PRETZEL MILKSHAKE

Ingredients
2 cups chocolate ice cream
4 fun-sized Snickers bars (or any chocolate bar of your choice)
1 package of pretzel sticks, broken up
Directions:
1. Add soft ingredients and mix with liquid as per recipe.
2. Blend until desired consistency is achieved. Add more liquid to make less thicker shakes.
3. Open lid and add toppings to introduce more textures (crunchy candy pieces, soft fruit, etc.)
4. Blend for 5-10 seconds more if you want additional ingredients mixed in.

MOCHA MINT MILKSHAKE

Ingredients
4 cups mint chocolate chip ice cream
½ cup chocolate syrup
½ cup cold strong coffee
½ cup milk
¼ cup chocolate syrup, for cup swirls
¼ cup chopped Andes mints
Whipped cream, for garnish
Directions:

1. Add soft ingredients and mix with liquid as per recipe.
2. Blend until desired consistency is achieved. Add more liquid to make less thicker shakes.
3. Open lid and add toppings to introduce more textures (crunchy candy pieces, soft fruit, etc.)
4. Blend for 5-10 seconds more if you want additional ingredients mixed in.

RED VELVET MILKSHAKE

Ingredients
4 scoops red velvet ice cream
1 cup of milk
3-4 drops red food coloring (optional)
whipped cream
peppermint candies, crushed
maraschino cherries
Directions:
1. Add soft ingredients and mix with liquid as per recipe.
2. Blend until desired consistency is achieved. Add more liquid to make less thicker shakes.
3. Open lid and add toppings to introduce more textures (crunchy candy pieces, soft fruit, etc.)
4. Blend for 5-10 seconds more if you want additional ingredients mixed in.

TOASTED MARSHMALLOW MILKSHAKE

Ingredients
5 scoops high-quality vanilla ice cream
2 tablespoons whole milk
1 tablespoon plain greek yogurt
5 jumbo toasted marshmallows (can toast in oven or over stove)
Whipped cream, for topping
Graham crackers, crushed, for garnish
Directions:
1. Add soft ingredients and mix with liquid as per recipe.

2. Blend until desired consistency is achieved. Add more liquid to make less thicker shakes.
3. Open lid and add toppings to introduce more textures (crunchy candy pieces, soft fruit, etc.)
4. Blend for 5-10 seconds more if you want additional ingredients mixed in.

COFFEE MILKSHAKE

Ingredients
1 cup cold-brewed coffee (see recipe below for instructions, or use strong brewed coffee that has been well chilled.)
4 giant scoops vanilla ice cream
1 tablespoon chocolate syrup plus extra for drizzling
whipped cream
Directions:
1. Add soft ingredients and mix with liquid as per recipe.
2. Blend until desired consistency is achieved. Add more liquid to make less thicker shakes.
3. Open lid and add toppings to introduce more textures (crunchy candy pieces, soft fruit, etc.)
4. Blend for 5-10 seconds more if you want additional ingredients mixed in.

MANGO MILKSHAKE

Ingredients
1 cup - chopped mango
2.5 cups - chilled milk
2 tsp - sugar (or as needed)
1 - green cardamom (optional)
ice cubes (optional)
Directions:
1. Add soft ingredients and mix with liquid as per recipe.
2. Blend until desired consistency is achieved. Add more liquid to make less thicker shakes.

3. Open lid and add toppings to introduce more textures (crunchy candy pieces, soft fruit, etc.)
4. Blend for 5-10 seconds more if you want additional ingredients mixed in.

MINT CHIP MILKSHAKE CUPCAKES

Ingredients
1 frozen, large banana
½ tsp pure vanilla extract
2 Tbsp melted coconut butter
½ to ⅔ cup milk of choice
Directions:
1. Add soft ingredients and mix with liquid as per recipe.
2. Blend until desired consistency is achieved. Add more liquid to make less thicker shakes.
3. Open lid and add toppings to introduce more textures (crunchy candy pieces, soft fruit, etc.)
4. Blend for 5-10 seconds more if you want additional ingredients mixed in.

ULTIMATE ICE CREAM SUNDAE MILK

Ingredients
1 Serving of Chocolate Syrup or Fudge (approx 2 Tbs)
3 Large Fresh Strawberries
1 Medium Ripe Banana
1 Serving of Vanilla Ice Cream or Frozen Yogurt (softened)
Chocolate Milk
Directions:
1. Add soft ingredients and mix with liquid as per recipe.
2. Blend until desired consistency is achieved. Add more liquid to make less thicker shakes.
3. Open lid and add toppings to introduce more textures (crunchy candy pieces, soft fruit, etc.)

4. Blend for 5-10 seconds more if you want additional ingredients mixed in.

CHOCOLATE COOKIE DOUGH MILKSHAKE

Ingredients
1 ¼ cups Chocolate Milk
5-6 scoops Cookie Dough Ice Cream
Chocolate Syrup
Whipped Cream
Cherries (optional)
Directions:
1. Add soft ingredients and mix with liquid as per recipe.
2. Blend until desired consistency is achieved. Add more liquid to make less thicker shakes.
3. Open lid and add toppings to introduce more textures (crunchy candy pieces, soft fruit, etc.)
4. Blend for 5-10 seconds more if you want additional ingredients mixed in.

25 DIY Whipped Natural Butters For Hair, Skin, and Body

Directions:
Body Butters & Creams:
1. Combine butter and oil ingredients in container and blend on medium until everything is blended smoothly (usually 25-45 seconds).
2. Add incense drops (if necessary) and blend for 1-5 seconds.
3. Re-blend as necessary.

HOMEMADE BODY BUTTER WITH SHEA AND COCONUT OIL

Ingredients
1/2 cup shea butter
1/4 cup coconut oil
1/4 cup olive or almond oil
10-15 drops essential oil, orange, or sandalwood
Directions:
Body Butters & Creams:
1. Combine butter and oil ingredients in container and blend on medium until everything is blended smoothly (usually 25-45 seconds).
2. Add incense drops (if necessary) and blend for 1-5 seconds.
3. Re-blend as necessary.

SKIN PERFECTING BODY BUTTER

Ingredients
2oz shea butter
2oz evening primrose oil
10 drops Young Living Jasmine oil
10 drops Young Living Frankincense oil
Directions:
Body Butters & Creams:

1. Combine butter and oil ingredients in container and blend on medium until everything is blended smoothly (usually 25-45 seconds).
2. Add incense drops (if necessary) and blend for 1-5 seconds.
3. Re-blend as necessary.

DREAMY HOMEMADE LEMON CREAM BODY BUTTER

Ingredients
6 tbsps coconut oil
¼ cup cacao butter
1 tbsp vitamin E oil
¼ teaspoon lemon essential oil
Directions:
Body Butters & Creams:
1. Combine butter and oil ingredients in container and blend on medium until everything is blended smoothly (usually 25-45 seconds).
2. Add incense drops (if necessary) and blend for 1-5 seconds.
3. Re-blend as necessary.

MANGO BODY BUTTER

Ingredients
1 cup shea butter
1/2 cup mango butter
1/2 cup almond oil
Mango essential oil (20-25 drops)
Directions:
Body Butters & Creams:
1. Combine butter and oil ingredients in container and blend on medium until everything is blended smoothly (usually 25-45 seconds).
2. Add incense drops (if necessary) and blend for 1-5 seconds.
3. Re-blend as necessary.

WHIPPED GINGERBREAD BODY BUTTER

Ingredients

1/2 cup Shea butter
¼ cup coconut oil
2 tbsp. almond oil
2 tsp or 2 Vitamin E capsules
2 tsp. Ground Ginger
1 tsp. Ground Cinnamon
1 tsp. Vanilla Extract
Directions:
Body Butters & Creams:
1. Combine butter and oil ingredients in container and blend on medium until everything is blended smoothly (usually 25-45 seconds).
2. Add incense drops (if necessary) and blend for 1-5 seconds.
3. Re-blend as necessary.

HOMEMADE BODY BUTTER BASE

Ingredients
1/2 cup each of organic
cocoa butter
shea butter
coconut oil
olive oil
1/2 teaspoon of essential oils
Directions:
Body Butters & Creams:
1. Combine butter and oil ingredients in container and blend on medium until everything is blended smoothly (usually 25-45 seconds).
2. Add incense drops (if necessary) and blend for 1-5 seconds.
3. Re-blend as necessary.

WHIPPED MOCHA BODY FROSTING

Ingredients
30g white cocoa butter
30g dark cocoa butter (or just more white cocoa butter)
60g shea butter or mango butter
40g olive oil (or other relatively plain liquid oil)

4 drops coffee essential oil
Directions:
Body Butters & Creams:
1. Combine butter and oil ingredients in container and blend on medium until everything is blended smoothly (usually 25-45 seconds).
2. Add incense drops (if necessary) and blend for 1-5 seconds.
3. Re-blend as necessary.

HONEY COCONUT BODY BUTTER

Ingredients
8g beeswax
36g virgin coconut oil
2 drops clove bud essential oil
25 drops labdanum essential oil
Directions:
Body Butters & Creams:
1. Combine butter and oil ingredients in container and blend on medium until everything is blended smoothly (usually 25-45 seconds).
2. Add incense drops (if necessary) and blend for 1-5 seconds.
3. Re-blend as necessary.

CRANBERRY BODY BUTTER

Ingredients
3 oz. refined shea butter
.25 oz. refined/deodorized cocoa butter
.2 oz. grape seed oil
.05 oz. pure tapioca starch
.1 oz. cranberry fragrance oil of choice
pinch coral oil locking mica shimmer, optional
Directions:
Body Butters & Creams:
1. Combine butter and oil ingredients in container and blend on medium until everything is blended smoothly (usually 25-45 seconds).
2. Add incense drops (if necessary) and blend for 1-5 seconds.

3. Re-blend as necessary.

ECZEMA RELIEF BODY CREAM

Ingredients
1/4 cup Shea butter
1/4 cup coconut oil
10 drops Lavender essential oil
5-10 drops Cedarwood essential oil
a few drops of vitamin E oil (optional)
Directions:
Body Butters & Creams:
1. Combine butter and oil ingredients in container and blend on medium until everything is blended smoothly (usually 25-45 seconds).
2. Add incense drops (if necessary) and blend for 1-5 seconds.
3. Re-blend as necessary.

WHIPPED SHEA BUTTER FOR HAIR & BODY

Ingredients
4 oz Raw shea butter, softened
6 tsp Virgin (unrefined) coconut oil, softened
4 tsp Castor oil
1 tsp Jojoba oil
8 tsp Aloe Vera Gel
Directions:
Body Butters & Creams:
1. Combine butter and oil ingredients in container and blend on medium until everything is blended smoothly (usually 25-45 seconds).
2. Add incense drops (if necessary) and blend for 1-5 seconds.
3. Re-blend as necessary.

BASIC BODY BUTTER

Ingredients
1-3/4 cups shea butter (unrefined is best)
1/2 cup coconut oil (extra virgin is best)
1/4 cup grapeseed oil

essential oils
Directions:
Body Butters & Creams:
1. Combine butter and oil ingredients in container and blend on medium until everything is blended smoothly (usually 25-45 seconds).
2. Add incense drops (if necessary) and blend for 1-5 seconds.
3. Re-blend as necessary.

COOLING ALOE AND MINT BODY LOTION

Ingredients
¼ cup grated beeswax
½ cup coconut oil
½ cup aloe vera gel, room temperature
⅛ teaspoon peppermint oil
Directions:
Body Butters & Creams:
1. Combine butter and oil ingredients in container and blend on medium until everything is blended smoothly (usually 25-45 seconds).
2. Add incense drops (if necessary) and blend for 1-5 seconds.
3. Re-blend as necessary.

PEPPERMINT BODY BUTTER

Ingredients
3 ounces pure cocoa butter
4 ounces coconut oil
4 drops peppermint essential oil
2 drops red food coloring
Directions:
Body Butters & Creams:
1. Combine butter and oil ingredients in container and blend on medium until everything is blended smoothly (usually 25-45 seconds).
2. Add incense drops (if necessary) and blend for 1-5 seconds.
3. Re-blend as necessary.

CHOCOLATE HAZELNUT BODY LOTION

Ingredients
14g cocoa butter
22g hazelnut oil
14g emulsimulse (or other complete emulsifying wax)
146 mL water
4g vegetable glycerin
1 blob/drop benzoin essential oil
2 drops cocoa absolute
Directions:
Body Butters & Creams:
1. Combine butter and oil ingredients in container and blend on medium until everything is blended smoothly (usually 25-45 seconds).
2. Add incense drops (if necessary) and blend for 1-5 seconds.
3. Re-blend as necessary.

WHIPPED WHITE CHOCOLATE BODY BUTTER

Ingredients
1/4 cup shea butter

1/4 cup cocoa butter

1/4 cup coconut oil

1/4 cup sweet almond oil

10-20 drops of essential oil
Directions:
Body Butters & Creams:
1. Combine butter and oil ingredients in container and blend on medium until everything is blended smoothly (usually 25-45 seconds).
2. Add incense drops (if necessary) and blend for 1-5 seconds.
3. Re-blend as necessary.

DOUBLE CHOCOLATE BODY BUTTER

Ingredients
1 cup cocoa butter (approximately 5 oz)
1/2 cup pure virgin coconut oil
1 tsp beeswax pastilles
2 tbsp almond oil
1 tbsp pure vanilla extract
1 1/2 tbsp raw cacao powder
Directions:
Body Butters & Creams:
1. Combine butter and oil ingredients in container and blend on medium until everything is blended smoothly (usually 25-45 seconds).
2. Add incense drops (if necessary) and blend for 1-5 seconds.
3. Re-blend as necessary.

HOMEMADE BABY SKIN CREAM

Ingredients
¼ cup cocoa butter (or 32 cocoa butter wafers)
¼ cup shea butter
2 tbsps olive oil
1 tbsp castor oil
Directions:
Body Butters & Creams:
1. Combine butter and oil ingredients in container and blend on medium until everything is blended smoothly (usually 25-45 seconds).
2. Add incense drops (if necessary) and blend for 1-5 seconds.
3. Re-blend as necessary.

HOMEMADE NOURISHING FACE CREAM

Ingredients
1/2 cup coconut oil
1/2 cup shea butter
1/4 cup of almond oil
5-6 drops of essential oil

Directions:
Body Butters & Creams:
1. Combine butter and oil ingredients in container and blend on medium until everything is blended smoothly (usually 25-45 seconds).
2. Add incense drops (if necessary) and blend for 1-5 seconds.
3. Re-blend as necessary.

HOMEMADE FACE LOTION

Ingredients
3 1/2 tbsp organic Shea butter

2 tbsps Jojoba oil

3 tbsps of Aloe Leaf Juice

4 drops lavender essential oil of choice

A pint sized mason jar
a small glass jar
Directions:
Body Butters & Creams:
1. Combine butter and oil ingredients in container and blend on medium until everything is blended smoothly (usually 25-45 seconds).
2. Add incense drops (if necessary) and blend for 1-5 seconds.
3. Re-blend as necessary.

WHIPPED PEPPERMINT BARK BODY BUTTER

Ingredients
¼ cup cocoa butter
¼ cup shea butter
¼ cup coconut oil
2 Tbs. vitamin E oil
¼ tsp. peppermint extract
Directions:
Body Butters & Creams:
1. Combine butter and oil ingredients in container and blend on medium until everything is blended smoothly (usually 25-45 seconds).
2. Add incense drops (if necessary) and blend for 1-5 seconds.
3. Re-blend as necessary.

BEACH BUTTER BALM

Ingredients
2 oz. Cocoa butter – Natural
2 oz. Shea butter – natural
2 oz. Monoi butter
1 tsp. Argan oil
3 tsp. Sweet almond oil
3 tsp. Aloe vera Gel
1/4 tsp. Vitamin E Natural
5 mL(s) Exotic coconut fragrance oil
Directions:
Body Butters & Creams:
1. Combine butter and oil ingredients in container and blend on medium until everything is blended smoothly (usually 25-45 seconds).
2. Add incense drops (if necessary) and blend for 1-5 seconds.
3. Re-blend as necessary.

PRETTY IN PINK BODY BUTTER

Ingredients
1 cup coconut oil
1 ½ cup vegetable shortening
1-3 drops pink food dye
5-10 drops essential oils (optional)
Directions:
Body Butters & Creams:
1. Combine butter and oil ingredients in container and blend on medium until everything is blended smoothly (usually 25-45 seconds).
2. Add incense drops (if necessary) and blend for 1-5 seconds.
3. Re-blend as necessary.

LEMON CREAM BODY BUTTER

Ingredients
6 tbsps coconut oil
¼ cup cacao butter
1 tbsp vitamin E oil
¼ teaspoon lemon essential oil
Directions:
Body Butters & Creams:
1. Combine butter and oil ingredients in container and blend on medium until everything is blended smoothly (usually 25-45 seconds).
2. Add incense drops (if necessary) and blend for 1-5 seconds.
3. Re-blend as necessary.

ULTRA HEALING FOOT CREAM

Ingredients

1/4 cup olive oil infused with calendula and chamomile
1/4 cup lavender infused coconut oil
1/4 cup cocoa butter
25g grated beeswax
25 drops peppermint essential oil
10 drops lemongrass essential oil
5 drops vanilla essential oil
5 drops tea tree essential oil
5 drops lavender essential oil
Directions:
Body Butters & Creams:
1. Combine butter and oil ingredients in container and blend on medium until everything is blended smoothly (usually 25-45 seconds).
2. Add incense drops (if necessary) and blend for 1-5 seconds.
3. Re-blend as necessary.

APPENDIX:RECIPES INDEX

WALNUT COCONUT MILK WITH TURMERIC AND CINNAMON 74
WATERMELON JUICE 50
WATERMELON RASPBERRY LIME JUICE 50
WATERMELON SMOOTHIE 38
WHIPPED GINGERBREAD BODY BUTTER 105
WHIPPED MOCHA BODY FROSTING 106
WHIPPED PEPPERMINT BARK BODY BUTTER 109
WHIPPED SHEA BUTTER FOR HAIR & BODY 107
WHIPPED WHITE CHOCOLATE BODY BUTTER 108
WINTER MINT CHOCOLATE PROTEIN SHAKE 29

Y

YELLOW CURRY POWDER 91
YOUTHBERRY WILD ORANGE BLOSSOM TEA BLEND 93

Z

ZA'ATAR SEASONING BLEND 91
ZIPPY LEMON PEPPER RUB 89

CPSIA information can be obtained
at www.ICGtesting.com
Printed in the USA
BVHW010337250221
600517BV00005B/53